David Paul Busuttil

The Molecular Basis of Glucose 6-Phosphate Dehydrogenase Deficiency

David Paul Busuttil

The Molecular Basis of Glucose 6-Phosphate Dehydrogenase Deficiency

From the Laboratory to the Clinic

LAP LAMBERT Academic Publishing

Imprint

Any brand names and product names mentioned in this book are subject to trademark, brand or patent protection and are trademarks or registered trademarks of their respective holders. The use of brand names, product names, common names, trade names, product descriptions etc. even without a particular marking in this work is in no way to be construed to mean that such names may be regarded as unrestricted in respect of trademark and brand protection legislation and could thus be used by anyone.

Cover image: www.ingimage.com

Publisher:
LAP LAMBERT Academic Publishing
is a trademark of
Dodo Books Indian Ocean Ltd. and OmniScriptum S.R.L publishing group

120 High Road, East Finchley, London, N2 9ED, United Kingdom
Str. Armeneasca 28/1, office 1, Chisinau MD-2012, Republic of Moldova, Europe
Managing Directors: Ieva Konstantinova, Victoria Ursu
info@omniscriptum.com

Printed at: see last page
ISBN: 978-3-659-76899-6

Zugl. / Approved by: London, University of London Royal Postgraduate Medical School, Diss., 1990/91

THE MOLECULAR BASIS OF GLUCOSE 6-PHOSPHATE DEHYDROGENASE DEFICIENCY AND THE CHARACTERISATION OF A NEW VARIANT: FROM THE LABORATORY TO THE CLINIC

David P Busuttil MD MRCP (UK) FRCP FRCPath

Dedicated to my niece Stephanie who, due to unforeseen circumstances, added a new dimension to my life.

TABLE OF CONTENTS

Page

ABSTRACT

The genomic DNA of a twelve year old Sardinian boy with a chronic haemolytic state due to G6PD deficiency was analysed. To identify the molecular lesion in the G6PD gene, exons II-XIII were amplified by PCR, followed by M13 cloning. Purified phage clones were sequenced by the Sanger dideoxy termination method using the universal primer or a set of oligonucleotides homologous to intron sequences near intron-exon junctions. 85% of the coding sequence of the G6PD gene was sequenced. One base difference from wild type G6P DB sequence was found – a C→ T transition at position 1318 in exon XI causing a substitution of leucine to phenylalanine at position 440. The amino acid substitution entails no net change in polarity and is consistent with the normal electrophoretic mobility of the enzyme. The drastic change of an aliphatic to an aromatic amino acid could disrupt the protein structure, adversely affecting its stability. The substitution occurs in a part of the protein which is conserved in G6PD from yeast, rat, *P. Falciparum*, *E. Coli* and *Drosophilia*, and is thought to be involved in the binding of NADP. It is a unique, as yet un-described mutation associated with CNSHA. The variant has been designated G6PD Telti.

INTRODUCTION

Function of G6PD in Erythrocytes
Structure of G6PD
Regulation of G6PD Activity
Clinical Manifestations of G6PD Deficiency
Public Health Significance of G6PD Deficiency
Mechanism of Haemolysis
Classification of G6PD Variants
Relationship between Variant G6PD and Clinical Expression
Polymorphism of G6PD
Inheritance of G6PD Deficiency
Developments in the Study of G6PD
The G6PD Gene
Aim of Project

Glucose-6-phosphate dehydrogenase (G6PD) deficiency is a multifaceted problem that is of interest to haematologists, biochemists, molecular biologists, pop ulation geneticists and malariologists.

Function of G6PD in erythrocytes

Glucose is the main energy source of the erythrocyte. After phosphorylation of glucose to glucose 6-phosphate (G6P) in the hexokinase section, two alternative pathways are available – the Embden-Meyerhof pathway that generates ATP and the hexose monophosphate pathway (HMP) shunt. G6PD catalyses the first step - the oxidation of G6P to 6 phosphoglucono lactone (6PG) by NADP, which is reduced to NADPH.

$$G6PD + NADP \xrightarrow{\text{G6PD}} 6PG + NADPH$$

In the normal, unstressed erythrocyte, approximately 10% of G6P is metabolised by way of the HMP pathway, while the other 90% follows the Embden -Myerhof pathway.

The most important function of the HMP pathway is to generate a supply of NADPH to maintain glutathione in the reduced state (GSH). In the steady state, 99.8% of glutathione is reduced and only 0.2% is in the oxidised form (GSSG). The generation of GSH is accomplished by the enzyme g lutathione reductase (GR) in which NADPH serves as a reducing agent.

$$GSSG + NADPH + H^+ \xrightarrow{\text{GR}} 2GSH + NADP$$

A variety of erythrocyte components have active sulphydryl (-SH) groups. These include enzymes e.g. hexokinase and GR, membran e proteins e.g. band 3, and haemoglobin. These –SH groups are maintained in the reduced form by the action of GSH.

The erythrocyte is vulnerable to oxidative damage as a result of its oxygen transport functions. Free oxygen radicals are produced by the di ssociation of molecular oxygen from oxyhaemoglobin. These radicals are converted to hydrogen peroxide (H_2O_2) by superoxide dismutase (SOD)

$$2O^{2-} + 2H^+ \longrightarrow H_2O_2 + O_2$$

The erythrocyte contains two enzyme systems that detoxify H_2O_2-
1) Glutathione Peroxidase: GSH is the substrate and in the process is oxidised to GSSG.
   $$2GSH + H_2O_2 \longrightarrow GSSG + 2H_2O$$
   The GSH is subsequently regenerated by glutathione reductase.
2) Catalase: The erythrocyte has abundant supplies of catalase which catalyses the inactivation of H_2O_2
   $$2H_2O_2 \longrightarrow 2H_2O + O_2$$
   NADPH is a structural component of catalase, there being four tightly bound NADPH molecules per catalase tetramer.

In normal erythrocytes, the contribution by the two systems is about equal; catalase however, does the job more efficiently due to a lower NADPH utilisation. [19]

Structure of G6PD

The active form of G6PD consists of a dimer or tetramer of identical subunits. These are in a pH dependant equilibrium with abo ut equal proportions at pH 7.2 - the physiological intracellular pH of the erythrocyte.

In vitro, the inactive monome rs associate to form active dime rs and tetramers in the presence of NADP. There are four tightly bound NADP molecules per tetr amer; indeed, the binding constant is too high to be measured, and they constitute, what is referred to as "structural NADP". The enzyme can bind four additional molecules of NADP with high affinity, which are referred to as "substrate NADP" and two molecules of NADPH. The NADP and NADPH compete for the same sites.

Regulation of G6PD activity

The regulatory step of HMP metabolism is the G6PD reaction.

In normal erythrocytes, the G6PD reaction proceeds at a rate much lower than the V_{max} of G6PD. The kinetic properties of G6PD explain t he low utilisation rate of G6PD. In resting cells, G6PD is markedly inhibited by NADPH and the normal level of NADP is well below the K_m of the enzyme. Furthermore, the level of G6P in normal erythrocytes is under that required for maximal G6PD activity and ATP at physiological concentration, is a competitive inhibitor of G6PD with respect to G6P. Let us consider the situation where a normal erythrocyte is exposed to an oxidant stress. The generation of O_2^- radicals and H_2O_2 will be countered by the oxidation of GSH to GSSG. The resulting availability of GSSG, will use up NADPH and increase the cellular level of NADP, in an attempt to maintain the pool of GSH. The reversal of the NADP:NADPH ratio releases the inhibition of G6PD and G6P is oxidised at a faster rate.

So, the healthy erythrocyte responds to the oxidant stress by increasing the activity of its HMP pathway. There is a vast reserve of reductive potential, since the normal erythrocyte operates at only 1-2% of its maximum potential. This reserve is substantially decreased in G6PD deficient cells, in which the defective enzyme operates much nearer its V_{max}.

Clinical manifestations of G6PD deficiency

G6PD deficiency is associated with a wide range of disease states.

1) Acute haemolytic anaemia(AHA) - The administration of certain drugs, ingestion of fava beans or infections can trigger acute haemolytic episodes, characterised by a reduction of circulating erythrocytes, jaundice, haemoglobinuria and a compensatory increase in the number of reticulocytes. These episodes vary in severity and duration. In the absence of haemolytic agents, there are no signs of deficiency.

2) Chronic non-spherocytic haemolytic anaemia(CNSHA) - This is the most severe consequence of G6PD deficiency. It occurs in the rarer individual s so severely deficient in G6PD enzyme, that they suffer from anaemia throughout their lives. Patients exhibit varying degrees of anaemia and *all* have a reticulocytosis (4-34%) even in the absence of oxidant stress. Unlike other congenital haemolytic anaemias, splenomegaly is rare [35] although gallstones may be present. Spherocytes are not seen in significant numbers in the blood film and the osmotic fragility is normal. It does not usually respond to splenectomy. The anaemia can increase in severity on administration of drugs or during infections.

3) Neonatal jaundice (NNJ) - jaundice appearing within one to four days of age is associated with many cases of G6PD deficiency. It occurs commonly

in the Mediterranean and Far East, but it is now a major problem in Africa and has been reported in blacks in North America.

The relative contribution of erythrocyte destruction and impaired hepatic function to the pathogenesis of NNJ are disputed. Impaired hepatic function, similar to that seen in normal premature infants may be a major cause. Some d istinctive features of neonatal erythrocytes may contribute to the degree of jaundice, e.g. increased ascorbic acid or decreased Vitamin E, glutathione reductase and catalase levels.

A striking feature is the wide variation in its frequency and severity i n different populations. For example, it is more common among Africans in Africa than among African resident in America. The same is true for Greeks in Greece compared to subjects of Greek ancestry in Australia.

Environmental and genetic factors are invok ed as an explanation for this heterogeneity.

G6PD in other tissues

G6PD is distributed in *all* cells [28]. A striking feature of G6PD deficiency is that there are usually no manifestations in other tissues. This is not surprising as the erythrocyte is unable to renew its supply of G6PD, on which it is uniquely dependent for survival. Other cells can replace the enzyme and may have alternative means of producing NADPH.

Granulocytes have a higher G6PD activity than other cells. This is explained by their great demand for NADPH in (1) the synthesis of membrane lipid for phagocytosis and (2) in the respiratory burst. So, it is remarkabl e that in most cases of severe G6PD deficiency, there is no clinical evidence of granulocyte dysfunction. Only 6 out of the 80 or so CNSHA variants are associated with infection. Common to all these cases is a complete absence of erythrocyte G6PD activity, less than 5% of normal enzyme activity in granulocytes and failure to undergo a respiratory burst . [43]

Public Health Significance of G6PD Deficiency

G6PD deficiency stands out among other enzymopathies in its public health significance.

1) It is the most common enzymopathy, estimated to affect 400 million people worldwide.[28].
2) It is the commonest red cell enzymopathy to caus e NNJ. The jaundice can be severe and if untreated may result in kernicterus. So, it is a preventable cause of mental retardation.
3) It is common in areas of the world where fava beans are a staple diet. Understanding the disease will prevent what is potenti ally the gravest consequence of G6PD deficiency- favism. Therefore, unlike most other genetic disorders, *its most adverse effects can be prevented*.

Mechanism of Haemolysis

1) <u>Drugs</u> – Several potentially haemolytic drugs are known to generate H_2O_2. In addition, some drugs may form free radicals that oxidise glutathione directly, without formation of H_2O_2 as an intermediate. In normal cells, after exposure to primaquine, the O_2- and H_2O_2 produced is effectively removed by glutathione peroxidise, so no damage o ccurs. In G6PD deficiency, the rate of operation of glutathione peroxidise is impaired, despite the accelerated rate of HMP metabolism, so that H_2O_2 is allowed to reach dangerous levels. This leads to oxidation of the –SH groups of protein 3, haemoglobin a nd glutathione. The complexing between the –SH groups of glutathione and of the other proteins, results in the formation of mixed disulphides, which are probably unstable and precipitate as Heinz bodies. Heinz bodies have been shown to consist of denatured globin chains, band 3, ankyrin, bands 4.1, 4.9 and 5; glycophorins A and B; and autologous IgG [1]. On passage through the spleen, they tend to be removed from the cell, leaving characteristic "bite marks". It is assumed that the associated part of the me mbrane is damaged and accounts for the intravascular haemolysis that has been universally accepted to operate in AHA.

Evidence is now accumulating that implicates a predominant extravascular destruction of erythrocytes. This is supported by signs of mas sive erythrophagocytosis in bone marrow and post -mortem examinations. The clustering of band 3 in the Heinz bodies is thought to enhance the binding of autologous anti -

band 3 IgG. The IgG coated erythrocytes are recognised by Fc receptors of macrophages and phagocytosis is triggered. Once bound, cluster ed anti-band 3 binds avidly to C3b, rendering the newly opsonised erythrocyte even more susceptible to phagocytosis.[1]

2) Fava beans – are rich in two glucosidic compounds – vivine and convicine, that generate pyrimidine aglycones - divicine and isouramil by the action of an enzyme present in the seeds, B -glucosidase. Aglycones have been implicated as the haemolytic agents. They are strong reducing agents that activate O_2 in the presence of GSH to form O_2- free radicals, and then H_2O_2 by SOD. In the process, the aglycones form oxidised intermediates that are recycled at the expense of GSH. The activity of glucosidase is very low in young seeds, increases to a maximum in ripe seeds and decreases again in older se eds. The variability in the levels of these components in the different cultivars together with the way the beans are consumed may account in part for the variability in clinical expression.

3) Infections – the mechanism of haemolysis is not known. It has be en proposed that the generation of H_2O_2 observed when leucocytes phagocyti se bacteria might be a source of damage to G6PD deficient cells. The influenza virus has been shown to preferentially lyse G6PD deficient cells *in vitro*. Similar effects may occur *in vivo*.[5]

4) Diabetic ketoacidosis (DKA) – is traditionally stated as being capable of precipitating haemolysis. This, however, is based on only six cases of black G6PD deficient subjects with inadequate documentation. A review of 36 episodes of DKA in G6PD deficient subjects yielded only 10 in whom haemolysis occurred and these were all associated with infection or drug administration. *Moreover, the presence of DKA in itself did not exacerbate the severity of the haemolytic episodes* [45].

In CNSHA, the residual G6PD activity is thought to be inadequate to detoxify H_2O_2, which is produced even under steady state conditions, leading to a considerable reduced erythrocyte life span. The red cell membrane has been shown to contain two types of high molecular weig ht aggregates - one type consisting of spectrin, the other of spectrin and other proteins, e.g. band 3, but not globins (therefore, they are not related to Heinz bodies). These aris e from the disulphide bridges (that would normally be prevented by GSH) bet ween spectrin molecules and between spectrin and other proteins. They decrease the cell defor mability and may do so suffi ciently to make it recognisable by macrophages as abnormal, thus leading to extravascular haemolysis.

It is probable that the anti-band 3-complement mediated erythrocyte removal is operative in CNSHA. IgG-coated erythrocytes are preferentially destroyed by the spleen, whereas the liver is the major site of phago cytosis of C3b-coated cells.[25] The predominance of the latter route of dest ruction, could explain the absence of splenomegaly in a substantial group of patients, the failure to demonstrate significant splenic sequestration and the poor response to splenectomy.[32]

Classification of G6PD variants

More than 400 variants have been described [3]. They are characterised by analysis of the enzyme properties, namely -
   i)   G6PD activity
   ii) Electrophoretic mobility
   iii) K_m G6PD and NADP
   iv) Utilisation of substrate analogues, 2 deoxy G6PD and amino NADP
   v)   Thermal stability
   vi) Optimal pH for enzyme activity

They have been classified into five classes according to the level of enzyme activity and their clinical manifestations.
Class I variants are associated with CNSHA
Class II variants are those with severe deficiency defined as activity less than 10% of normal. The prototype of this class is G6PD Mediterranean.
Class III variants are those with moderate deficiency, having 10-60 % of normal residual activity. The prototype of this class is G6PDA.
Class IV variants are those with enzyme activity within the nor mal range e.g. G6PDA and B.
Class V variants have increased activity compared to normal.

   -   The latter two classes have increased activity compared to normal.
   -   All variants associated with AHA are in classes II and III, but the reverse does not hold.

Relationship between variant G6PD and clinical expression

Two features determine whether a G6PD variant will cause AHA or CNSHA.

1) The residual activity of the enzyme.
2) The kinetic properties – Analysis of kinetic data reveals that variants in Class II often have abnormally high substrate affinities (low K_m) for G6PD or NADP or both, whereas variants in Class I tend to have high K_m for substrates i.e. they utilise the substrate poorly. Furthermore, K_i NADPH is significantly decreased (i.e. greater affinity for the inhibitor) in 35% of Class I variants.

G6PD is the main controller of erythrocyte NADP and NADPH levels. For instance, when the affinity for NADP is decreased, less NADP is utilised, so the NADP level will be sustained. This will offer more substrate to G6PD, thus compensating for the lowered affinity. Similarly, if the enzyme binds more avidly to NADPH, less NADPH will be available to inhibit G6PD in the cell.

By contrast, the level of G6P depends on hexokinase activity and on glycolysis. It can be kept relatively constant by vast reservoirs of plasma glucose.

Thus, the residual enzyme activity and the K_m for G6PD are the most important factors determining whether a variant is associated with AHA or CNSHA [27].

Polymorphism of G6PD

G6PD is a polymorphic enzyme. Deficiency is frequent in three main geographic regions, namely W. Africa (and hence the US), the Mediterranean, Middle East and South East Asia. These are areas where malaria is or was at one time, common. This has led to the suggestion that the enzyme-deficient subject has a selective advantage by being relatively resistant to malaria, as illustrated by the following example - Amongst the Farsi-Zorastrian population in the great salt desert of Iran, living at high altitude in a dry malaria-free area, the incidence of G6PD deficiency is low (1%). In members of the same ethnic group, who migrated 1,000 years before to the W. coast of India, a region hyperendemic for malaria, the incidence is much higher (17%), possibly as a result of natural selection.[2]

The selection hypothesis was supported by studies on females heterozygous for G6PD A⁻ that showed a higher degree of infestation of normal cells, than that of G6PD deficient cells (Luzzatto and Usanga 1967). *In vitro*, G6PD deficiency inhibits growth of the malarial parasite, possibly by causing oxidative injury to the parasite.

Parasites that survive passage through G6PD deficient red cells become adapted to the deficient cells after several cycles. The mechanism of adaptation is not yet known, but it is proposed that the parasite can induce synthesis of its own G6PD[30]. Studies of plasmodium G6PD and of the gene encoding it are in progress[48]. Since hemizygous and homozygous individuals have only G6PD deficient cells, they are not protected. The advantage conferred by G6PD appears to be limited to female heterozygotes, as the mixed population of normal and deficient cells interferes with the process of adaptation.

The geographic distribution of G6PD deficiency closely parallels that of the fava bean. This is surprising as one would have expected the enzymopathy to be excluded in such areas due to the negative effect on favism on survival. It has been suggested that the effect of fava beans may actually enhance the beneficial effect of G6PD in mitigating malarial infections. The aglycones may act as natural antimalarial compounds interfering with the intraerythrocyte development of the parasite. In this regard, they may be more effective in G6PD deficient than in normal cells [14,20]. This may explain the patchy distribution of G6PD deficiency in malaria endemic areas.

A variant is polymorphic, when its frequency in at least one population is more than 1%. They are not found in Class I. A variant is said to be sporadic when only one or very few cases have been identified. Sporadic variants cannot be allowed to increase in frequency in a population, even in the face of positive selection, in view of the relatively severe disadvantage they entail.

Figure 1.   Distribution map of G6PD deficiency.

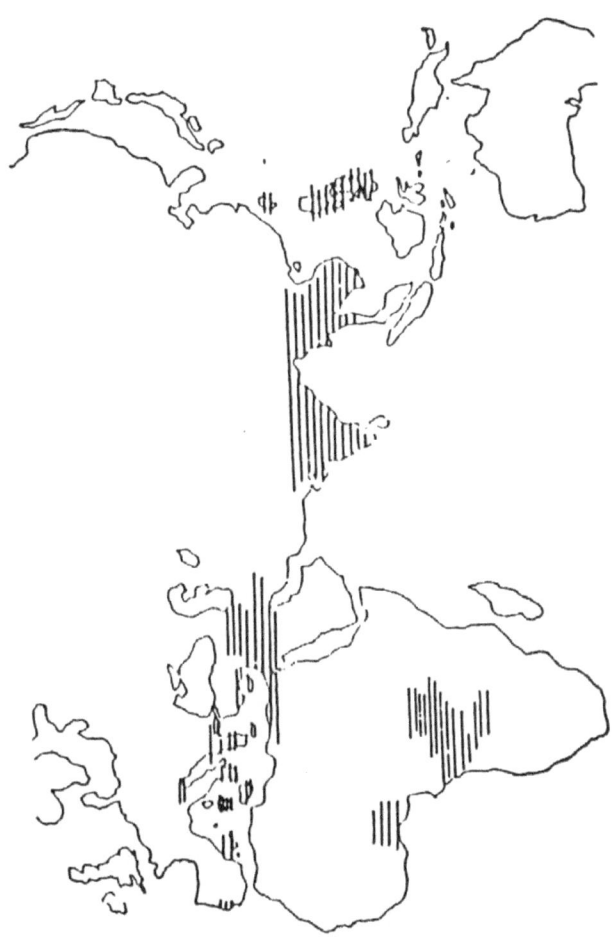

Inheritance of G6PD deficiency

The gene for G6PD is located on the X-chromosome. The defect is fully expressed in the male hemizygote and female homozygote. In terms of clinical expression, it is sometimes classified as X-linked recessive. This is not true as it is *partially* expressed in heterozygous females. Because of the phenomenon of X-chromosome inactivation, heterozygotes have two populations of erythrocytes - normal and deficient, which vary in proportion. The larger the size of the deficient population, the greater the susceptibility to haemolysis.

Developments in the study of G6PD

Over the past decade, there has been some confusion concerning the significance of the gradually increasing number of putative variants characterised by their biochemical properties.

It soon became apparent that standardisation of the techniques would be needed if lab to lab comparison of the variants was to be meaningful. A committee for the WHO recommended standard techniques for the biochemical characterisation of G6PD variants in 1967.

Despite standardisation, many ambiguities remained. Since enzymes are unstable, side by side comparison was not possible, differences in the properties of different batches of reagents and minor variations in technique between laboratories (even when it was thought that standards were being followed) were common. G6PD Cornell is a classic example of how inter-laboratory differences of the biochemical properties of the same variant can occur. Characterised as a unique variant, it was later found that the propositus was a member of the same large family from which G6PD Chicago had originally been described[4]. The reported characteristics of these enzymes are rather dissimilar, yet based on genetic evidence, G6PD Cornell and Chicago must be the same.

Determining the molecular structure of G6PD was the solution. Sequencing of G6PD protein has been extremely difficult, because of the small quantity available, even from normal blood. The breakthrough came in 1986 when Persico et al cloned the G6PD gene and determined the cloning sequence .[34]

The G6PD gene

The G6PD gene is 18 kb long and consists of 13 exons and 12 introns. The coding exons vary in size from 38bps (exon III) to 695 bps (exon XIII). Exon I is non-coding. The introns are all smaller than 1kb, except intron II, which is 11 kb[31].

A binding site for pyridoxal phosphate has been identified in exon VI. A peptide with an almost identical sequence has been found in yeast G6PD and it contains a lysine residue that is essential for enzyme activity in the organism [26]. The binding of pyridoxal 5-phosphate to human G6PD produces substantial inactivation. G6PD prevents loss of activity, suggesting that this part of the enzyme may be essential for the binding of G6P or at least for maintaining the G6P binding site in the correct conformation.[13]

Aim of Project

With improved methods of DNA cloning and sequencing, it has now become possible to determine rapidly and reliably the specific alteration in the DNA sequence. The aim of the project was to analyse genomic DNA of a known G6PD deficient subject.

Table 1. The genomic organisation of the G6PD gene.

Exons	bp	Introns	bp
I	60 (60)		
		IVS 1	550
II	128 (8)		
		IVS 2	11 kb
III	38		
		IVS 3	95
IV	109		
		IVS 4	550
V	218		
		IVS 5	573
VI	159		
		IVS 6	180
VII	126		
		IVS 7	400
VIII	94		
		IVS 8	450
IX	187		
		IVS 9	140
X	236		
		IVS 10	100
XI	77		
		IVS 11	103
XII	93		
		IVS 12	97
XIII	695 (607)		

CASE REPORT

The propositus was a 12 year old boy from Telti, a village on Sardinia. He was admitted after falling ill with passage of dark urine. On examination, the only positive finding was moderate splenomegaly. He had a haemoglobin of 9.9g/dl, haematocrit of 29% and reticulocyte count of 7.9%. Transfusion was withheld and he was kept under observation for 15 days. His past history was reassessed.

He weighed 2.7 kg at birth and suffered from neonatal jaundice. Within a nine year period he had seven hospitalisations for moderate to severe haemolytic crisis, characterised by fever, prostration, jaundice and haemoglobinuria. These occurred in response to drug administration (sulphonamides and paracetamol on one occasion), viral infections and sometimes without any obvious cause. The haemoglobin tended to fall within the 5.2-9.2 g/dl range, the reticulocyte count rising into the 4.5-24.3% range, with the serum bilirubin elevated up to 6.83 mg/dl. Repeated blood transfusions were required.

On day 15 post-crisis, his haematological profile was assessed. Investigations revealed a mild anaemia (Hb 11.3 d/dl), haematocrit 37%, red cell count 3.95 x 10^6, a reticulocytosis of 9.5%, normal blood indices (MCV 93; MCH 28.6; MCHC 30.1), an elevated serum bilirubin (2.2mg/dl and serum ferritin 469 mg/ml. The G6PD level was 0.4u/g (normal value 6.73+/- 2-10) with an electrophoretic mobility of 100%. The leucocyte and platelet counts were normal. The hap toglobin level was 48.6mg/dl (normal value 30-200mg/dl). The acidified glycerol lysis test was normal and the pyruvate kinase assay was non-specifically elevated. A diagnosis of CNSHA was made.

Haematological studies on the mother revealed a mild anaemia (Hb 11.4 mg/dl, Hct 39.7%) and a reticulocyte count of 2.1%. The G6PD level was reduced at 3.4 u/g (normal value 6.73+/-2.1). Other investigations including blood indice s, serum ferritin, haptoglobin (180 mg/dl) and acidified glycerol lysis test were norm al. The HbA_2 level was 4.65%.

Figure 2. Topographical map of Sardinia.

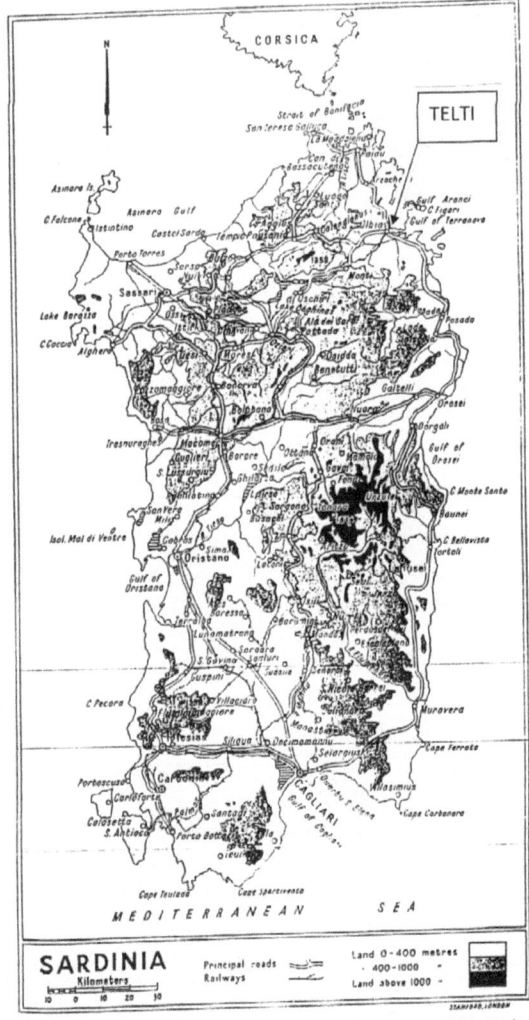

MATERIALS

Enzymes
M13 as the vector
E.Coli as the host
Agarose gel electrophoresis
Polyacrylamide gel electrophoresis
Sephadex filtration columns

Enzymes

<u>Restriction endonucleases</u>
Restriction endonucleases have a protective role in bacteria by degrading foreign DNA of, for instance, an infecting bacteriophage. They cleave DNA only if it contains a specific recognition sequence. The cell protects its own DNA by methylating A or C residues within the recognition sequence.

Type II restriction enzymes are used in DNA cloning. They cleave DNA *within* the recognition sequence. The length of the recognition sequences varies between four and six residues and the sequence is usually rotationally symmetrical.

They cleave DNA leaving a phosphate group on the newly created 5' end and a hydroxyl group at the 3' end. When an enzyme cleaves the recognition site at the centre of symmetry, it generates blunt ends. If an enzyme cuts off centre, it creates two fragments with overlapping ends. These are called sticky ends as base pairing between them can stick the DNA molecule together again.

Table 2   **Recognition sequences of Restriction enzyme**

Enzyme	Sequence	Termini
Xba I	↓ 5' - T C T A G A - 3' 3' - A G A T C T - 5' ↑	Sticky
Eco RI	↓ 5' - G A A T T C - 3' 3' - C T T A A G - 5' ↑	Sticky
Xho I	↓ 5' - C T C G A G - 3' 3' - G A G C T C - 5' ↑	Sticky
Sma I	↓ 5' - C C C G G G - 3' 3' - G G G C C C - 5' ↑	Blunt
Sal I	↓ 5' - G T C G A C - 3' 3' - C A G C T G - 5' ↑	Sticky

T4 Ligase

T4 ligase is purified from *E. Coli* that has been infected with T4 phage. Within the cell, it carries out the important function of repairing any breaks in the DNA strand.

It catalyses the joining of a 5'-phosphate and a 3'-hydroxyl group to generate a phosphodiester bond. It can join together two restriction fragments, provided they share the same sticky or blunt ends. Ligation of compatible sticky ends is efficient as they can base pair with one another by hydrogen bonding, forming a relatively stable structure for the enzyme to work on. Ligation of blunt ends is not so efficient as the ligase is unable to "catch hold" of the molecule and has to wait for chance associations to bring the ends together. A higher enzyme concentration is therefore used. The reaction is ATP dependent.

In the ligation reaction, the vector ends lie a relatively short distance apart and will find each other more frequently than a target molecule, so the tendency would be for re-circularisation of the vector, without joining to the target molecule.

Calf Intestinal phosphatise (CIP)

CIP removes 5' phosphate groups from a DNA fragment to generate a hydroxyl end. It is used after digestion of the vector, to prevent the ends from rejoining as the 5'hydroxyl group is not a substrate for ligase.

T4 Polynucleotide Kinase

T4 kinase is derived from *E.Coli* infected with T4 phage. It has a reverse effect to CIp, adding phosphate groups to the 5'end. A de-phosphorylated vector will ligate to a target DNA molecule only if the latter can provide a phosphate group, hence the use of Y4 kinase in phosphorylating the blunt ends of target DNA. The reaction is ATP dependent.

DNA Polymerase I

DNA polymerase synthesises a new strand of DNA complementary to an existing template in the presence of a primer. It is endowed with nuclease activity degrading the existing strand as it synthesises the new one. The polymerase and nuclease activities are controlled by different parts of the enzyme molecule and can be separated. The polymerase part is called the Klenow fragment. It has two uses (1) to generate radiolabelled DNA probes (2) to generate single stranded DNA in the dideoxy sequencing method.

In sequencing, resolution has now been improved by the use of sequenase, a chemically modified bacteriophage polymerase. It incorporates dNTP's and ddNTP's at a more consistent rate, creating a more even pattern.

<u>Taq polymerase</u>

Taq polymerase was isolated from the thermophilic bacteria *Thermus aquaticus* from a hot spring of Yellowstone National Park 20 years ago. The substitution of Taq polymerase for the previously used DNA polymerase I Klenow fragment has permitted automation of PCR. Formerly, PCR involving Klenow enzyme required moving the samples manually between two sources - one at 95^0C for denaturation and one at 37^0C, necessitating the addition of fresh enzyme during each cycle. Since Taq polymerase can withstand repeated exposure to high temperature the inconvenience of having to add fresh enzyme during each cycle is avoided. Automation has permitted the use of three distinct temperatures. The temperatures for annealing and extension can now be optimised independently. This has significantly increased the specificity and yield of the reaction. The higher temperature optimum of Taq Polymerase (T_m of 75-80^{0}C) has allowed the use of higher temperatures for annealing and extension, thereby, minimising the extension of mismatched primers. At 37^0C many of these mismatched primers were sufficiently stable to be extended by the Klenow enzyme resulting in non-specific products.

After a certain number of cycles, the amplification product gradually stops accumulating exponentially and enters the plateau phase for a number of reasons -(1) gradual inactivation of Taq polymerase (2) substrate excess as a result of having synthesized more DNA than the amount of enzyme present in the mix (3) competition by non-specific amplification products for the limiting enzyme (4) Re-association of the single stranded PCR products before the annealed primers can be extended.

Taq polymerase is sensitive to the concentration of magnesium(Mg $^{2+}$) in the buffer. Excess Mg^{2+} results in accumulation of non-specific amplification products and insufficient Mg^{2+} reduces the reaction yield.

M13 as the vector

M13 is a single-stranded phage packed in a filamentous protein coat. The phages attach to F.pili of *E. Coli* and are therefore able to infect only male cells.

The phage contains one circular single-stranded DNA molecule - the (+) strand approximately 6,500 nucleotides in length. Once inside the cell, the strand acts as the template for the synthesis of a complementary strand- the (-) circular replicating form, RF, which can be isolated and is used as a double stranded cloning vector.

After 100-200 copies per cell of the RF have accumulated, M13 synthesis becomes asymmetric producing large amounts of only the (+) strand. These are eventually incorporated into protein coats and are continually extruded from the infected cells.

Although the cells are not lysed by the M13 infection, their growth is somewhat inhibited. Thus, an M13 plaque appears as a turbid area in which cells are growing more slowly than the surrounding uninfected cells. The main advantage of M13 as a cloning vector is that *genes are obtained in a single stranded form*. They can be used as templates for Sanger dideoxy sequencing.

The essential requirement for a cloning vector is that it has a means of replicating in the host cell. Except for a 507 nucleotide region known as the intergenic sequence (IS), the rest of the genome consists of ten closely packed genes essential for replication. In the M13 derivatives constructed as cloning vectors, two types of sequences have been inserted into the IS, without affecting phage liability -

1) A fragment of the *E.Coli* Lac gene consisting of the regulatory region and the N-terminal end of the B-galactosidase gene. The N-terminal part of the B- galactosidase protein produced is able to complement the product of a defective B-galactsidase gene in the host cell. This complementation produces active B-galactosidase which gives rise to blue plaques when the phage and cells are grown in the presence of the inducer IPTG and the chromogenic substrate x-gal.

2) A DNA fragment containing several unique restriction sites that has been inserted into the B-galactosidase gene. This fragment, known as the polylinker or multiple cloning site (MSC) does not affect the ability of the B-galactosidase product to complement the defective B - galactosidase of the host cell. However, insertions of foreign DNA into the region destroys the complementation. Recombinant phages give rise to colourless plaques

when grown in the presence of IPTG and X-gal. This forms the basis of a simple, quick chromogenic test to identify recombinant plaques.

An oligonucleotide that is complementary to the region of M13 adjacent to the MCS can be synthesized. This serves as a primer for Sanger dideoxy sequencing of *any* DNA insert. It is called the universal primer. It obviates the need of having to make a different primer for each individual fragment of cloned DNA to be sequenced.

Figure 3.   Structure of M13 mp10 cloning vector.

GAATTC GAGCTCGCCCGGGGATCC TCTAGA GTCGAC CTGCAGCCCAAGCTT

EcoRI	SstI		BamHI	Xbal	Sal I	Pst I	Hind III
MP10		Smal, Xmal			Acc I,		
					Hincll		

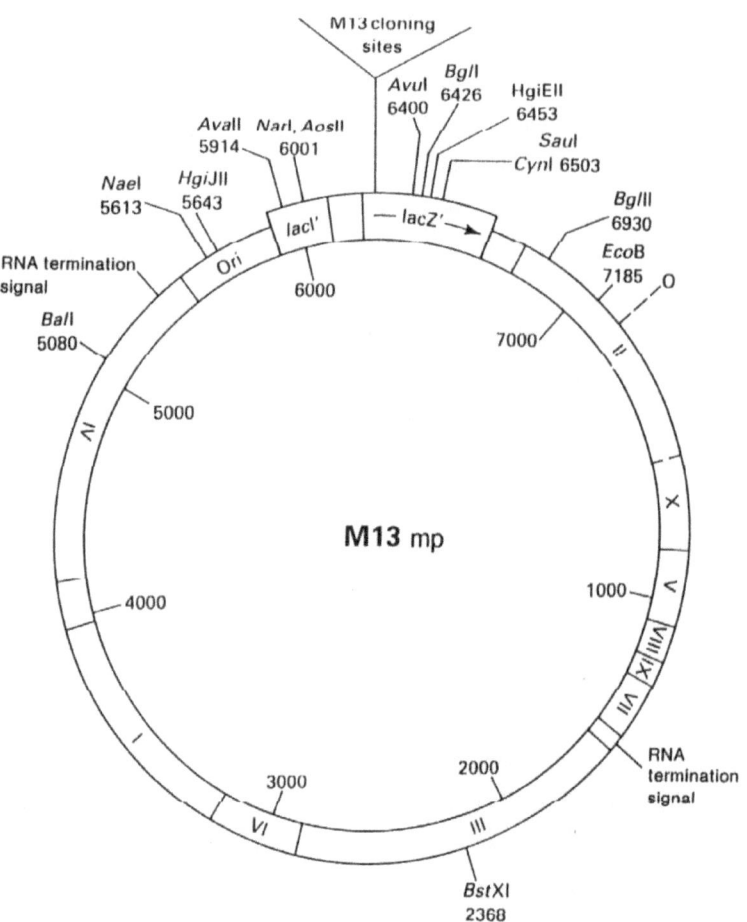

E. Coli as the host organism

The JM101 strain of *E. Coli* is a "safe vector" that has been genetically engineered to disable it in such a way that it cannot grow well outside the test tube. This is to prevent recombinant molecules with the potential for causing disease from escaping to the environment.

The strain used in M13 cloning has the following genotype -JM 101(lac,pro)thi-1F[pro AB$^+$,lac Iq,lac Z(M15)],Tra D36] in which

1) The genes for proline biosynthesis and lactose catabolism are deleted.
2) The thiamine biosynthesis gene is inactivated. To grow this strain, the growth medium must be supplemented with these nutrients, which it cannot synthesize or process.
3) The F-factor has-
   i An artificial prolene biosynthesis gene inserted
   ii Deletion of the regulator B-galactosidase gene lac Iq
   iii A deletion of the N-terminal part of the lac ZB-galactosidase gene resulting in the formation of a defective galactosidase called the M15 protein.
   iv The Tra D mutation that decreases its frequency of replication.

Agarose gel electrophoresis

Agarose is a highly purified polysaccharide derived from agar. When it polymerises by the formation of hydrogen and hydrophobic bonds, it creates a complex system of pores through which DNA molecules can migrate.

Agarose gel electrophoresis is the standard method use d to separate, identify and purify DNA fragments. The location of DNA within the gel can be determined as bands of DNA stained with the dye ethidium bromide (which intercalates between the base pairs) fluoresce a bright orange when viewed under ultraviolet light. As little as 1 ng of DNA can be detected.

The gel is submerged in buffer and the DNA samples are loaded into wells within the gel. For loading, DNA is mixed with a solution containing a tracking dye (to tell how far the samples have migrated) and a weighing agent (to ensure the sample sinks

33

into the well). An electric field is applied across the gel. As nucleic acids have a negative charge, they migrate to the anode. The migration rate depends on four factors:

1) The molecular size of DNA.
2) The agarose concentration, which determines the pore size. The higher the concentration, the smaller the pore size , the lower the migration.
3) The conformation of the DNA- closed circular (supercoil) DNA migrates fastest followed by the nicked circular form, and slowe st is the linear form. Under some conditions the order is reversed.
4) The applied current- at low voltages, the rate of migration of linear DNA is proportional to the voltage applied.

Polyacrylamide gel electrophoresis

A polyacrylamide gel is capable of re solving single-stranded oligodeoxynucleotides 300-500 bases in length, which differ in size by a single deoxynucleotide. Its important application is in sequencing.

Acrylamide monomers polymerise into long chains by the addition of ammonium persulphate and tetramethyl-ethylene diamine (TEMED) which serve as the initiator and catalyst respectively for the reaction. These polymers are the covalently linked by a cross-linker –N,N'-methylene-bis-acrylamide that actually holds the gel together. Urea is incorporated in the gel to denature the DNA molecules. The electrophoresis is carried out at a high voltage to ensure the strands do not re -associate.

Each band in the gel contains only a small amount of DNA, so autoradiography must be used to visualise the resul ts. For this purpose ^{35}S is preferred to ^{32}P. Due to the lower energy of the decay particles of the ^{35}S isotope, the bands are sharper, there is less radiolysis of DNA, less background on the autoradiograph and it is intrinsically safer. The 88-day half-life compared to 14 days of ^{32}P also means that it has a longer shelf-life and is therefore more economical if used over a long period.

Sephadex filtration columns

Sephadex is a bead-forming gel prepared by cross-linking dextran with epichlorohydrin. The large number of hydroxyl groups renders the gel extremely hydrophilic. Consequently, sephadex swells considerably in water and electrolyte solutions. The G- types of sephadex differ in their degree of cross -linking and hence fractionation range.

As a solute passes down a chromatographic column, its movement depends on the bulk flow of the mobile phase and upon the Brownian movement of the solute molecules, which causes their diffusion both into and out of the stationary phase. The separation of the components depends on the different abilities of the molecules to enter pores that contain the stationary phase. Very large molecules which never enter the stationary phase move through the chromatographic bed fastest. Smaller molecules which can enter the gel pores move more slowly since they spend a proportion of their time in the stationary phase.

Sephadex columns have been used to remove from DNA preparations the free nucleotides and other types of smaller molecules which may interfere with subsequent manipulation e.g. removal of the ^{32}P-labelled nucleotides not incorporated into the probe.

METHODS

PCR
Treatment of PCR products
Preparation of M13 vectors
Ligation
Preparation of competent *E.Coli*
Transfection of *E. Coli*
Identification of recombinant clones
Preparation of single-stranded M13 template
Sequencing

PCR

The Polymerase chain reactions (PCR) were set up as follows:

DNA	3ul
Primer 1(0.1ug/ul)	5ul
Primer 2(0.1ug/ul)	5ul
10 x cetus buffer[1]	10ul
dNTP's (10mM)	3ul
H_2O	74ul

A negative control with no template DNA was set up with each batch to detect potential contamination. The reagents were mixed and denatured at 94 ^{0}C in the PCR machine for 10 minutes. 5ul of diluted Taq Polymerase (diluted to 0.5 u/ul in 1 x Cetus buffer) was added to each tube and the reaction run through 30 cycles in the PCR machine. Each cycle consisted of:

45 seconds denaturing at 94^{0}C
1 minute annealing at 56^{0}C
1 minute extension at 72^{0}C (3 minutes for Exon X-XIII) followed by a 10 minute extension at 72^{0}C at the end of the run.

---

[1] 10 x Cetus buffer is 0.1M Tris pH 8.3;0.5M KCL; 12 mM $MgCl_2$; 0.1% gelatine; 0.5% NP40; 0.5% Tween 20

Figure 4.   PCR of G6PD exons

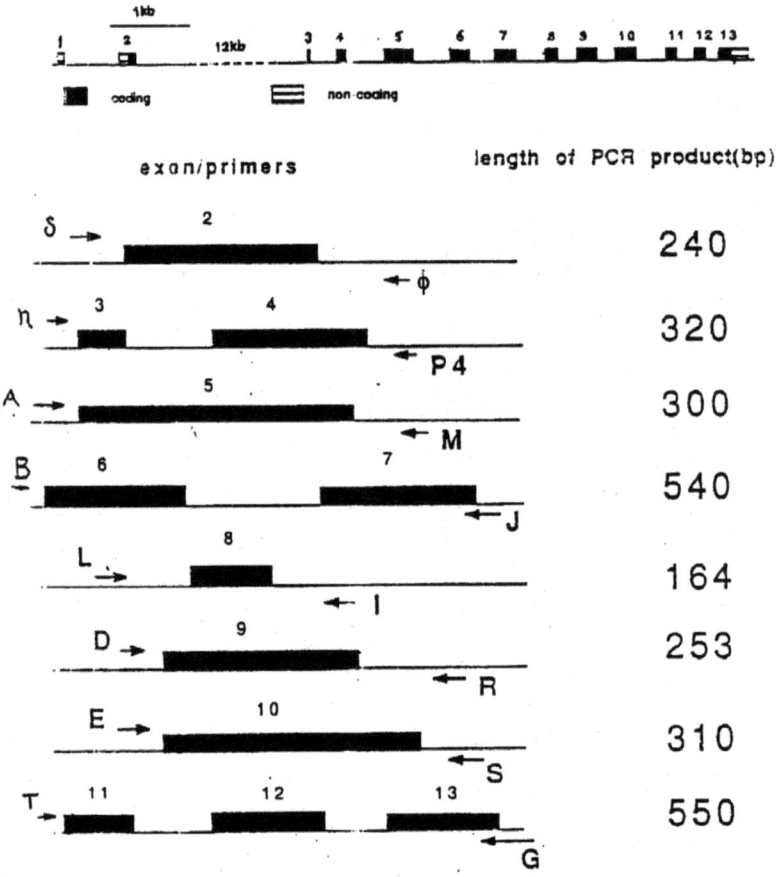

exon/primers   length of PCR product(bp)

δ →   2   240

η → 3   4   320
                         P4

A →   5   300
                    M

B → 6   7   540
                      J

L →   8   164
              I

D →   9   253
                      R

E →   10   310
                    S

T → 11   12   13   550
                    G

38

Table 3   G6PD OLIGOS USED FOR PCR (5' -> 3')

δ   CTCTAGAAAGGGGCTAACTTCTCAA

φ   GGAATTCCTGGCTTTTAAGATTGGG

η   CAGCCACTTCTAACCACACACCT

P4   CCGAAGTTGGCCATGCTGGG

A   CTGTCTGTGTGTCTGTCTGTCC

M   GGCCAGCCTGGCAGGCGGGAAGG

B   ACTCCCCGAAGAGGGGTTCAAGG

J   CCAGCCTCCCAGGAGAGAGGAAG

L   GGAGCTAAGGCGAGCTCTGGC

I   GGCATGCTCCTGGGGACTGTG

D   CAAGGAGCCCATTCTCTCCCTT

E   CTGAGAGAGCTGGTGCTGAGG

S   AGGCCGCCCACCCTCCACACT

T   GCAGGCAGTGGCATCAGCAAG

G   GGGAAGGAGGGTGGCCGTGG

K   GAGGCTCCTGAGTACCACCC

PCR Products

1. Purification- either (1) by phenol extraction followed by Sephadex G50 fractionation or (2) purification from a gel.
2. Enzymatic manipulation
   i) Templates with sticky ends were digested using the following protocol:

Purified DNA	50ul
10 x RE buffer	50ul
Restriction enzyme	1ul
H_2O	43ul
Total volume	100ul

The reactions were incubated at $37\,^0C$ for 4 hours

   ii) Templates with blunt ends were phosphorylated as follows;

Purified DNA	15ul
10 x kinase buffer[2]	3ul
10mM ATP	3ul
H_2O	30ul
T4 polynucleotide kinase	0.5 ul

The reaction was incubated for $37\,^0C$ for 1 hour.

---

[2] 10 x Kinase buffer is 500 mM Tris pH 7.6; 100mM $MgCl_2$; 50 mM DTT; 1 mM spermidine; 1 mM EDTA

Figure 5. Graphical representation of restriction sites of PCR fragments.

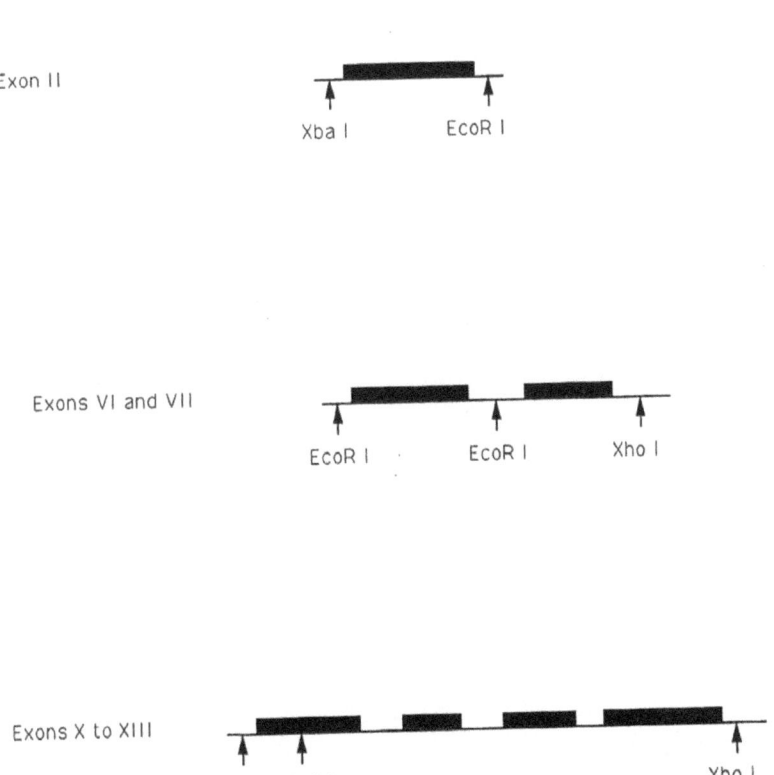

Exon II

Xba I   EcoR I

Exons VI and VII

EcoR I   EcoR I   Xho I

Exons X to XIII

Xho I   Pst I   Xho I

41

3. <u>Phenol extraction</u> – phenol denatures and precipitates protein thereby inactivating enzymes that could interfere with subsequent manipulation. An equal volume of phenol was added to the reaction mixture, which was vortexed and microfuged for 1 minute. Two layers separate out, with nucleic acids in the upper aqueous layer and the proteinaceous material forming a white layer at the interface. The upper layer was pipette d out and placed in a new tube.

4. <u>Ethanol precipitation</u> – permits the concentration of DNA into a small volume. In the presence of the monovalent cation e.g. Na^+ and at a temperature of -20^0C or less, absolute ethanol efficiently precipitates polymeric nucleic acids. It has the added advantage of leaving monomeric nucleic acids in solution.

To the reaction mixture, one tenth the volume of 3M sodium acetate and three volumes 100% ethanol was added. The reagents were mixed well and left at -70^oC overnight.

The mixture was microfuged for 10 minutes and the supernatant removed. The pellet was washed with 150ul of 70% ethanol and microfuged for 5 minutes. The supernatant was again removed, the pellet left to dry at room temperature and then dissolved in 25ul of water.

Preparation of M13 Vectors

1. <u>Digestion</u> – The digestion reactions were set up as follows:

M13 mp 10 DNA(2.2 ug/ml)	2ul
10 x buffer	2ul
Restriction enzyme	2ul
H_2O	14ul
Total volume	20ul

The reactions were left at $37\,^{0}$C overnight except the Sma I reaction, which was left at room temperature. In cases when two enzymes were used, 1ul of each was used.

      2. <u>Dephosphorylation</u> – To the previous reaction mix were added :

10 x CIP[3]	4ul
CIP	2ul
H_2O	14ul

To attain a final volume of 40 ul. The mix was incubated at $37\,^{0}$C for 2 hours.

      3. Phenol extraction + Sephadex G50 fractionation

Ligation

The ligation reactions were set up as follows for each template:

Tube	M13	PCR fragment	H_2O	Ligase mix
1	1ul	-	4ul	5ul
2	1ul	0.5ul	3.5ul	5ul
3	1ul	3ul	1ul	5ul

With an overnight incubation at $4\,^{0}$C

The ligase mix was as follows:

	Sticky ends	Blunt ends
5 x ligase buffer[4]	8ul	12ul
H_2O	11.5 ul	14ul
T4 ligase	0.5ul	4ul
Total	20ul	20ul

---

[3] 10 x CIP is 100mM Tris/HCL pH9.5;10mM spermidine; 1mM EDTA
[4] 5 X ligase buffer is 250mM Tris/HCL pH 7.6; 50mM $MgCl_2$, 10 mM ATP;10mM DTT; 5% Peg 8,000.

Table 4 - Summary of ligation reactions

	PCR Fragment	M13 mp10
I I	XbaI, EcoR1	XbaI, EcoR1
III,IV	blunt	Sma I
V	blunt	Sma I
VI,VII	EcoR1,Xho I	EcoR1, Sal I
VIII	blunt	Sma I
IX	blunt	Sma I
X-XII	Pst I, Xho I	Pst I, Xho I

Preparation of Competent *E.Coli*

5ml of SOB[5] medium was inoculated with JM101 and grown overnight at 37 ^{0}C.

The next day, the overnight culture of JM101 was diluted 1:100 with SOB and grown at 37^{0}C with shaking. The O.D. 600nm was regularl y checked, keeping in mind that the O.D. doubles in a 20 minute period. The growth was arrested when the O.D. reached 0.45 0.5, by chilling a 50ml aliquot in ice for 10 minutes.

---

[5] SOB medium contains 20% tryptone; 0.5% yeast extract;10mM MgCl $_2$; 10mM Mg 804.

The aliquot was centrifuged at 2,000rpm for 10 minutes at $4\,^0$C, the supernatant poured off and the pellet thoroughly drained.

The pellet was resuspended in 16.6 ml of transformation buffer (TFB) [6] by gentle vortexing and incubated on ice for 15 minutes.

The cell suspension was centrifuged again at 2,000 rpm at $4\,^0$C for 10 minutes, the supernatant poured off and the pellet thoroughly drained. The pellet was resuspended in 4 ml of TFG by gentle vortexing.

140ul of DD (consisting of DMSO and DTT) was squirted into the centre of the cell suspension and the tube swirled for several seconds. The cell culture was incubated in ice for 10 minutes. Another 140ul aliquot of DD was added and the suspension was incubated in ice for another 10 minutes.

Transfection of *E.Coli*

Transfection refers to the uptake by a cell of a DNA molecule. Under normal conditions, *E. Coli* takes up only a limited amount of DNA. The $CaCl_2$ treated cells are said to be competent as they have an increased tendency to transform. The mechanism is not understood, but the ionic composition of TFB, at $4\,^0$C seems to enhance the binding of foreign DNA to the outside of the cell wall.

The actual uptake of DNA into the competent cells is stimulated by briefly raising the temperature to 42^0C. The mechanism of heat shock is not understood, but treatment of the cells with dimethylsulphoxide and diothiothreitol increases the permeability of the cell wall.

Two YT top agar was melted in a microwave ovem, left to cool and placed in a 55^0C waterbath for later use.

200ul of the competent JM101 suspension was pipetted into appropriately labelled 10 ml plastic tubes on ice. 5ul of each ligation was added to the respective aliquot, mixed and incubated on ice for 30 minutes.

---

[6] TFB is 10mM KCL ;45mM $MnCl_2$ $4H_2O$; 10mM $CaCl_2$-$2H_2O$; 3mM HA $CoCl_3$; 10mM K-MES. Final pH is 6.2+/- 0.1.

The cell culture was heat shocked by placing the tubes in a $42\,^0C$ water bath for 120 seconds and then put in ice again.

To each tube 10ul IPTG and 10ulX-Gal(2% in dimethyl formamide) was added. 4 ml of warm top agar was then added and the suspension poured (leaving 1 ml in the tube) onto the 2YT[7] plates.

A dilution was set up for each culture in order to obtain widely spaced plaque colonies. This was achieved by adding 100 ul of a JM 101 culture in exponential growth to the remaining 1ml of the suspension and topping up with 4ml of warm 2YT before pouring on the plates.

The plates were left to set for 10 minutes and then incubated at $37\,^0c$ overnight upside down, to prevent the condensation on the top plate from dripping onto the agar, thereby disseminating the colonies.

Identification of the recombinant clones

The next day the number of blue and white colonies on each plate were counted. The plates were incubated for one hour at $40\,^0C$.

"Hybond" disc filters were gently laid on top of the agar using fine forceps. There was no firm contact between plaques and filter, so that only unpackaged phage DNA molecules present in the plaques bind to the filter. Asymmetrical orientation marks were made by stabbing through the filter and into the agar with a needle.

The filters were peeled off with forceps, one at a time. They were laid to dry colony side up on a sheet of dry 3MM Whatman paper and labelled according to the plate number with waterproof ink.

The filters were sandwiched between two sheets of dry 3MM paper and baked at $80\,^0C$ in a vacuum oven. Baking fixes single stranded phage molecules to the filter through their sugar-phosphate backbones, so the bases are free to pair with complementary nucleic acids.

---

[7] 2YT contains 16g bactotryptone;10g yeast extract; 5g NaCl;1.5g agar –(w/v)

The master plates were stored upside down at $4\,^0C$ to stop cell growth and to prevent growth of mould.

1. Prehybridisation

The filters were floated on 2 x SSC^8 in a sandwich box. This prewashing step removes any absorbed medium or loose bacterial debris from the filters.

The filters were placed in a plastic bag, sealed along three sides and 25 mls of pre-warmed pre-hybridisation solution[9] added. The bubbles were removed and the last side of the bag sealed. The filters were incubated with agitation in a $65\,^0C$ water bath for 2-4 hours. Pre-hybridisation ensures that sites on the filter that can bind DNA non-specifically become saturated by unlabelled components in the pre-hybridisation solution.

2. Preparation of oligo-labelled probe:

1ml of the template (50ng/ul) derived from wild type G6PD cDNA together with 30ul of H_2O was pipetted into a screw-cap Eppendorf. It was denatured by boiling for 5 minutes and promptly chilled on ice.

The following reagents were added -

Commercial buffer solution (containing dNTP's) 10ul
Primer 5ul
Klenow enzyme 2ul
^{32}P dCTP 2ul

and incubated for one hour at $37\,^0C$.
The radioactive probed was eluted from a spinning sephadex column.

---

[8] 1 x SCC is 0.15M NaCl; 0.05M Na citrate
[9] Prehybridisation solution is 5 x SSPE; 5 x Denhardt's solution; 0.1% SDS; 5mg/ml denatured single stranded DNA. 20 x SSPE is 3.6M NaCL; 200 mM Na H_2PO_4 pH 7.4; 20mM EDTA pH 7.4
100 x Denhardt's solution is 2% polyvinylpyrrolidine; 2% Ficoll; 2% BSA(bovine serum albumen).

3.Hybridisation

The radioactive probe was denatured again by boiling for five minutes and chilling on ice thereafter.

A corner of the plastic bag was cut, the pre-hybridisation solution poured off and replaced with the same volume of pre-warmed pre-hybridisation solution.

The denatured probe was added, bubbles removed, the bag sealed and incubated overnight at 65^0C with agitation to ensure uniform exposure of the filters to the probe.

4.Washing

The next day, the bag was opened and emptied into a sink used for radioactive waste disposal. The filters were transferred to a sandwich box containing a pre-warmed washing solution of 3 x SSC, 0.1% SDS and swirled around to wash away excess unbound probe. The washing solution was then decanted into the sink.

The washing solution was added again to the filters and incubated with agitation for 15 minutes at 65^0C.

The solution was decanted and a second pre-warmed washing solution of 0.2 x SSC, 0.1% SDS was added and the filters were incubated with agitation for 15 minutes at 65^0C.

The filters were then placed on a Whatman 3 MM paper to dry at room temperature. The radioactivity incorporated into the filters was checked using a Geiger counter.

The filters were then placed between two sheets of Saran wrap, marked asymmetrically with fluorescent tape markers and exposed to an X-ray film with an intensifying screen in a cassette at -70^0C overnight.

4.Isolation of recombinant M13

5mls of 2YT medium was inoculated with a colony of JM 101 and grown overnight at 37^0C with shaking.

The next day, the overnight JM 101 culture was diluted 1 in 100 with 2YT and 2 ml aliquots were pipetted into 10 ml plastic tubes.

The autoradiograph was developed. Using the "hot spots" on the film, the orientation marks on the replica filters and master plates, the recombinant white plaques were identified. A single positive plaque was picked up with a yellow tip and dipped into the dilute JM 101 culture, one at a time.

The cultures were grown at 37^0C with shaking for 5-6 hours. Overgrowing can result in cell lysis and contamination with bacterial DNA.

Preparation of Single-Stranded M13 Template

The cultures were decanted into a 1.5ml Eppendorf and centrifuged for 3 minutes.

The supernatant was decanted in one continous movement so as not to transfer any cells into a new tube.

200ul of PEG/NaCl[10] was added, mixed well and left at room temperature for 15 minutes. Cloudiness was seen to appear.

The mixture was microfuged for 5 minutes, the pellet drained well, re-spun for 20 seconds and all the supernatant removed with a yellow tip. Any PEG/NaCl left over could inhibit the sequenase reaction.

The pellet was re-suspended in 100 ml TE by pipetting in and out with a yellow tip.

---

[10] PEG/NaCl is 20% polyethylene glycol; 2.5M NaCl. PEG is a long chain polymeric compound which in the presence of NaCl absorbs water, thereby causing macro molecular assemblies such as phage particles to aggregate. The PEG precipitate may also contain a certain amount of unwanted bacterial debris which can be removed by phenol extraction.

Phenol extraction was performed to dissolve the protein coat of the phage followed by ethanol precipitation.

Sequencing

The sequencing reactions were done for five reactions using the sequenase kit.

To 7 ul DNA in a 1.5 Eppendorf , 3ul of mix 1 was added.
Mix 1 contains 6ul primer[11], 12 ul reaction buffer[12]

The tubes were suspended in a 250 ml beaker containing water at 65 ^{0}C which was left to cool until the temperature fell below 30 ^{0}C. As the temperature slowly falls, it passes through the optimal range required for annealing of primer to template.

While the annealing step was in progress, four tubes were labelled G,A,T,C. To the bottom of each of the appropriate tubes, 2.5 ul of the termination mixes ddGTP, ddATP, ddTP and ddCTP were added.

The annealed template-primer was microfuged for three seconds and chilled on ice.

A second mix was set up:

0.1M DTT[13]	6ul
dGTP labelling mix[14]	2.4 ul
^{35}S d ATP	3ul
H_2O	9.6ul
Reaction buffer	10.6ul
Sequenase	1.4ul

5.5ul of the mix was added to each tube on ice mixing carefully at each step by pipetting up and down in a new tip. The reaction mixture was left at room temperature for five minutes.

---

[11] The universal primer GTAAAACGACCGGCCAGT or primers specific to a particular exon were used.
[12] Reaction buffer is 1000mM Tris HCL pH8.5; 50 mM $MgCl_2$
[13] Dithiothreitol is a reducing agent which helps keep the enzyme active.
[14] dGTP labelling mix contains 0.5 mM of all four types of dNTP's

3.5ul of the reaction mixture was added to the pre-warmed dideoxy nucleotides in the respective tubes and incubated at 37^0C for 5 minutes. The reactions were terminated by adding 4ul stop solution [15].

A 6% sequencing gel containing a 0.5 x TBE-2.5 x TBE gradient was prepared as follows:

	0.5 x gel mix	0.5 x gel mix
40% acrylamide[16]	150ml	150ml
10 x TBE	50ml	250ml
Urea	460g	460g
Bromophenol	-	50g
TEMED	140ul	40ul
Ammonium persulphate	140ul	40ul

The reaction mixes were denatured by heating between 80-100^0C for 5 minutes and loaded on the sequencing gel. It was run at 1800V until it warmed up and then at 45W until the bromophenol blue dye reached the bottom.

The gel was fixed for 15 minutes in 10% in 10% methanol 10% acetic acid and dried in a vacuum heater at 80^0C for one hour. The gel had to be completely dry, as an undried gel absorbs most of the radioactive emissions from the DNA bands.

The gel was exposed to an X-ray film overnight.

The film was developed and the sequences read against the normal G6PD sequence.

---

[15] Stop solution contains 100ml formamide (a denaturing agent), 0.1g bromophenol blue; 0.1g xylene cyanol; 2ml 0.5M Na2 EDTA

[16] 40% acrylamide consists of 380g acrylamide and 20g of N1N1 methylene bisacrylamide dissolved in 1 of H20.

RESULTS

PCR

PCR of the individual exons was performed. A 5ml aliquot of the resulting PCR reaction was analysed on a 1.2% minigel in 0.5 x TBE [17] run at 100V. The remaining products were stored at -20°C.

Figure 6 shows a typical PCR result. One track of Taq 1 digested p EMBL8+ was included on each gel as molecular weight markers(1443,1008, 613, 358, 278,193,108). By plotting a calibration curve of marker size against distance run, it was possible to determine the approximate sizes of the PCR fragments. The observed length was then matched against the expected length.

Figure 6: PCR of exons X-XIII

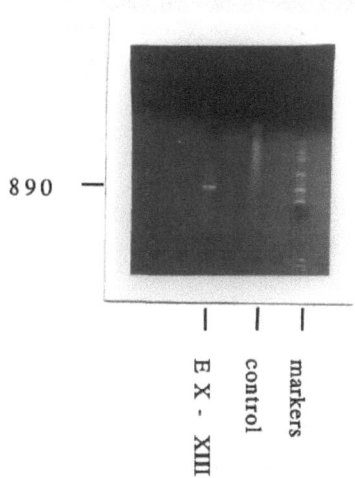

890 —

E X - XIII   control   markers

---

[17] 0.5 x TBE is 45mM Tris/HCL pH8; 45mM boric acid; 1 M EDTA

Purification of PCR Products

The PCR products were purified from a 1% agarose minigel in 1 x TAE [18] run at 50V. Under UV light the desired DNA, as represented by the thin band in the figure was spliced out. The DNA was then extracted using the Gene -Clean or Mermaid kit.

Figure 7

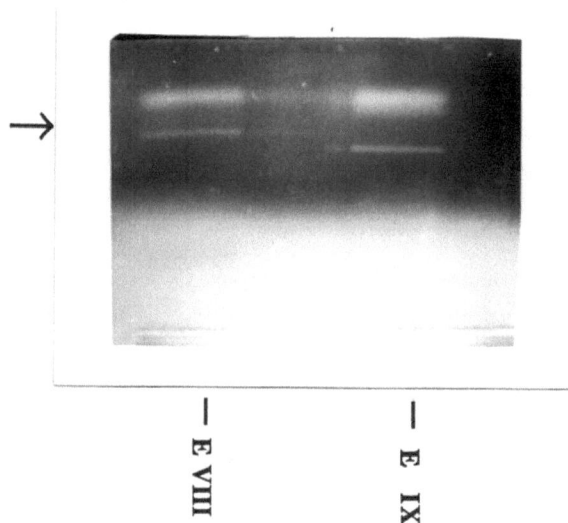

| E VIII | E IX |

Preparation of M13 Vectors

The M13 vectors were digested with respective restriction enzyme. 1ul of the resulting mix was analysed on a TBE mini gel run at 25V. Undigested DNA exists as a supercoil (s.c.) or in the "relaxed" form – open circle (o.c.).When digested, it assumes a linear form(l)

In figure 8,
Lane 1 shows partially cut M13 after EcoR1 digestion. Supercoil and linear forms are present.
Lanes 2 and 3 show M13 in linear form after SmaI and Sal I digestion respectively.
Lane 4 shows uncut M13 control in s.c. and o.c. configuration.

Figure 8.

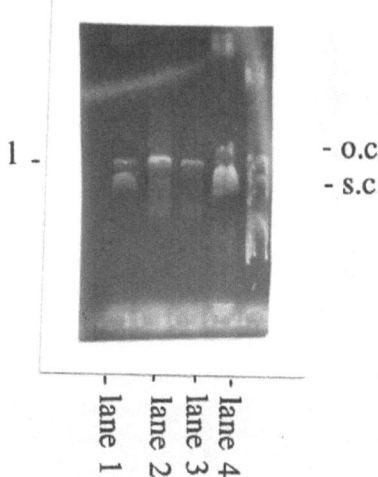

Identification of Recombinant Clones

The hybridised filters were exposed to an X-ray film overnight and the film developed. Figure 9 demonstrates hybridised colonies on the filters.

Figure 9.

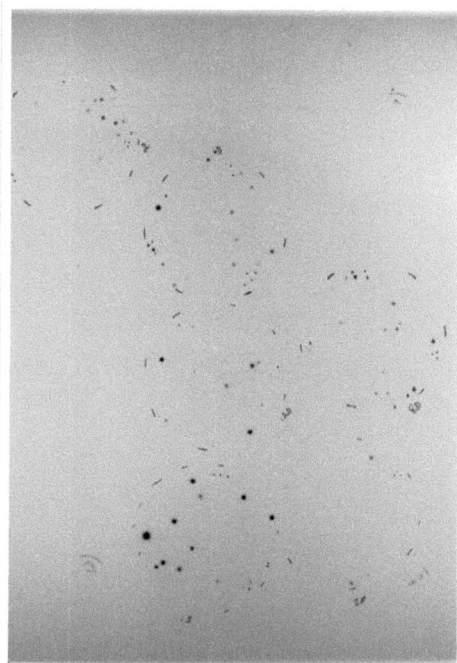

Preparation of Single-Stranded M13 Template

Single-stranded M13 was prepared. One fifth of the resulting solution was loaded on a 0.5% TBE minigel to assess quality and yield of the template as shown in figure 10.

Figure 10

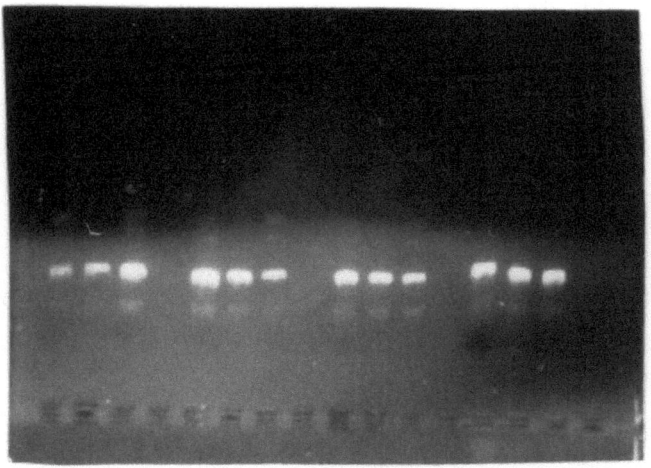

Sequencing

The coding sequence of the G6PD gene is shown. The highlighted areas were sequenced.

```
1   /   1                                    31   /   11
ATG GCA GAG CAG GTG GCC CTG AGC CGG ACC CAC GTG TGC GGG ATC CTG CGG GAA GAG CTT
met ala glu gln val ala leu ser arg thr his val cys gly ile leu arg glu glu leu
61   /   21                                   91   /   31
TTC CAG GGC GAT GCC TTC CAT CAG TCG GAT ACA CAC ATA TTC ATC ATC ATG GGT GCA TCG
phe gln gly asp ala phe his gln ser asp thr his ile phe ile ile met gly ala ser
121   /   41                                  151   /   51
GGT GAC CTG GCC AAG AAG AAG ATC TAC CCC ACC ATC TGG TGG CTG TTC CGG GAT GGC CTT
gly asp leu ala lys lys lys ile tyr pro thr ile trp trp leu phe arg asp gly leu
181   /   61                                  211   /   71
CTG CCC GAA AAC ACC TTC ATC GTG GGC TAT GCC CGT TCC CGC CTC ACA GTG GCT GAC ATC
leu pro glu asn thr phe ile val gly tyr ala arg ser arg leu thr val ala asp ile
241   /   81                                  271   /   91
CGC AAA CAG AGT GAG CCC TTC TTC AAG GCC ACC CCA GAG GAG AAG CTC AAG CTG GAG GAC
arg lys gln ser glu pro phe phe lys ala thr pro glu glu lys leu lys leu glu asp
301   /   101                                 331   /   111
TTC TTT GCC CGC AAC TCC TAT GTG GCT GGC CAG TAC GAT GAT GCA GCC TCC TAC CAG CGC
phe phe ala arg asn ser tyr val ala gly gln tyr asp asp ala ala ser tyr gln arg
361   /   121                                 391   /   131
CTC AAC AGC CAC ATG AAT GCC CTC CAC CTG GGG TCA CAG GCC AAC CGC CTC TTC TAC CTG
leu asn ser his met asn ala leu his leu gly ser gln ala asn arg leu phe tyr leu
421   /   141                                 451   /   151
GCC TTG CCC CCG ACC GTC TAC GAG GCC GTC ACC AAG AAC ATT CAC GAG TCC TGC ATG AGC
ala leu pro pro thr val tyr glu ala val thr lys asn ile his glu ser cys met ser
481   /   161                                 511   /   171
CAG ATA GGC TGG AAC CGC ATC ATC GTG GAG AAG CCC TTC GGG AGG GAC CTG CAG AGC TCT
gln ile gly trp asn arg ile ile val glu lys pro phe gly arg asp leu gln ser ser
541   /   181                                 571   /   191
GAC CGG CTG TCC AAC CAC ATC TCC TCC CTG TTC CGT GAG GAC CAG ATC TAC CGC ATC GAC
asp arg leu ser asn his ile ser ser leu phe arg glu asp gln ile tyr arg ile asp
601   /   201                                 631   /   211
CAC TAC CTG GGC AAG GAG ATG GTG CAG AAC CTC ATG GTG CTG AGA TTT GCC AAC AGG ATC
his tyr leu gly lys glu met val gln asn leu met val leu arg phe ala asn arg ile
661   /   221                                 691   /   231
TTC GGC CCC ATC TGG AAC CGG GAC AAC ATC GCC TGC GTT ATC CTC ACC TTC AAG GAG CCC
phe gly pro ile trp asn arg asp asn ile ala cys val ile leu thr phe lys glu pro
721   /   241                                 751   /   251
TTT GGC ACT GAG GGT CGC GGG GGC TAT TTC GAT GAA TTT GGG ATC ATC CGG GAC GTG ATG
phe gly thr glu gly arg gly gly tyr phe asp glu phe gly ile ile arg asp val met
781   /   261                                 811   /   271
CAG AAC CAC CTA CTG CAG ATG CTG TGT CTG GTG GCC ATG GAG AAG CCC GCC TCC ACC AAC
gln asn his leu leu gln met leu cys leu val ala met glu lys pro ala ser thr asn
841   /   281                                 871   /   291
TCA GAT GAC GTC CGT GAT GAG AAG GTC AAG GTG TTG AAA TGC ATC TCA GAG GTG CAG GCC
ser asp asp val arg asp glu lys val lys val leu lys cys ile ser glu val gln ala
901   /   301                                 931   /   311
AAC AAT GTG GTC CTG GGC CAG TAC GTG GGG AAC CCC GAT GGA GAG GGC GAG GCC ACC AAA
asn asn val val leu gly gln tyr val gly asn pro asp gly glu gly glu ala thr lys
961   /   321                                 991   /   331
GGG TAC CTG GAC GAC CCC ACG GTG CCC CGC GGG TCC ACC ACC GCC ACT TTT GCA GCC GTC
gly tyr leu asp asp pro thr val pro arg gly ser thr thr ala thr phe ala ala val
1021   /   341                                1051   /   351
GTC CTC TAT GTG GAG AAT GAG AGG TGG GAT GGG GTG CCC TTC ATC CTG CGC TGC GGC AAG
val leu tyr val glu asn glu arg trp asp gly val pro phe ile leu arg cys gly lys
1081   /   361                                1111   /   371
GCC CTG AAC GAG CGC AAG GCC GAG GTG AGG CTG CAG TTC CAT GAT GTG GCC GGC GAC ATC
ala leu asn glu arg lys ala glu val arg leu gln phe his asp val ala gly asp ile
1141   /   381                                1171   /   391
TTC CAC CAG CAG TGC AAG CGC AAC GAG CTG GTG ATC CGC GTG CAG CCC AAC GAG GCC GTG
phe his gln gln cys lys arg asn glu leu val ile arg val gln pro asn glu ala val
1201   /   401                                1231   /   411
TAC ACC AAG ATG ATG ACC AAG AAG CCG GGC ATG TTC TTC AAC CCC GAG GAG TCG GAG CTG
tyr thr lys met met thr lys lys pro gly met phe phe asn pro glu glu ser glu leu
1261   /   421                                1291   /   431
GAC CTG ACC TAC GGC AAC AGA TAC AAG AAC GTG AAG CTC CCT GAC GCC TAC GAG CGC CTC
asp leu thr tyr gly asn arg tyr lys asn val lys leu pro asp ala tyr glu arg leu
1321   /   441                                1351   /   451
ATC CTG GAC GTC TTC TGC GGG AGC CAG ATG CAC TTC GTG CGC AGC GAC GAG CTC CGT GAG
ile leu asp val phe cys gly ser gln met his phe val arg ser asp glu leu arg glu
1381   /   461                                1411   /   471
GGC TGG CGT ATT TTC ACC CCA CTG CTG CAC CAG ATT GAG CTG GAG AAG CCC AAG CCC ATC
ala trp arg ile phe thr pro leu leu his gln ile glu leu glu lys pro lys pro ile
1441   /   481                                1471   /   491
CCC TAT ATT TAT GGC AGC CGA GGC CCC ACG GAG GCA GAC GAG CTG ATG AAG AGA GTG GGT
pro tyr ile tyr gly ser arg gly pro thr glu ala asp glu leu met lys arg val gly
1501   /   501                                1531   /   511
TTC CAG TAT GAG GGC ACC TAC AAG TGG GTG AAC CCC CAC AAG CTC TGA
phe gln tyr glu gly thr tyr lys trp val asn pro his lys leu OPA
```

The mutation

A single base change was found in exon II - a C→T transition at position 1318 resulting in the substitution of leucine to phenylalanine. The mutation was demonstrated in five different clones.

Figure 11

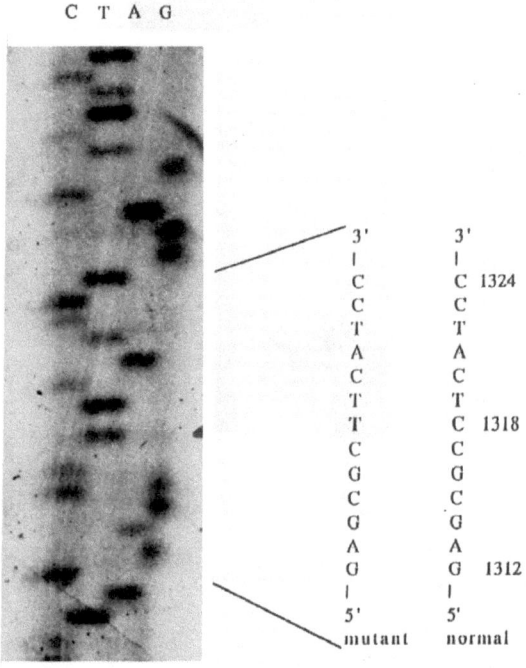

Comparison of mutant sequences of five different clones of exon XI with the normal sequence. There is a C →T transition at position 1318.

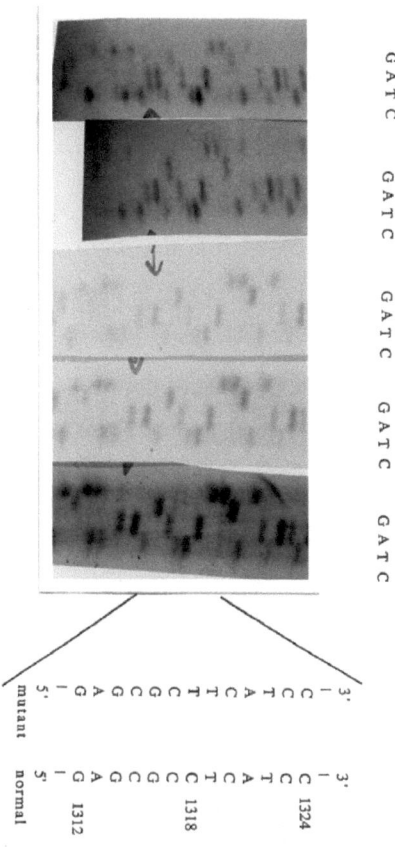

DISCUSSION

Molecular Basis of G6PD deficiency
Characterisation of a new variant

Molecular basis of G6PD deficiency

All variants described are due to point mutations. Four different variants contain two amino acid changes compared to normal G6PD B. However, these can be considered as single point mutations that have arisen in a G6PD A gene, a non - deficient variant common in African populations. G6PD is a *housekeeping gene*, present in all species so far tested, in which a change other than a point mutation may result in complete loss of function and death. This contrasts with the situation in other genes e.g. factor VIII and globin, where sizeable deletions are possible as complete loss of function may be compatible with survival.

The application of cloning and sequencing techniques has proved that biochemical characterisation of variants is misleading as was feared. Variants t hat were thought to be unique have proved to be identical at molecular level e.g. G6PD Matera, G6PD Betica, G6PD Alabama, G6PD Tepic, and G6PD Castilla were all found to be identical to the African variant G6PD A$^{-202A/376G}$. Likewise, what seemed to be alike in biochemical characterisation ended up being different. While in 90% of G6PD A - cases the second mutation is at nucleoside 202, the second mutation can also be at nucleotide 680(G→T) or at nucleotide 968 (T→C). [9]

Identification of the amino acid substitutions provides a powerful tool for understanding how the structure of G6PD relates to its function, as illustrated by the following case. A variant - G6PD Walter Reed was described which was unusual in that it exhibited no activity after purification, but became reactivated in the presence of NADP. It required high concentrations of NADP to maintain stability but it had a normal affinity for substrate NADP (normal K$_m$). This was in keeping with previous observations that there are two separate binding sites for "structural" and for "catalytic" NADP. It was proposed that G6PD Walter Reed had an abnormal binding site for "structural NADP".[11]

Table 5. Variants of Glucose-6-Phosphate Dehydrogenase.

VARIANT	NUCLEOTIDE SUBSTITUTION	AMINO ACID SUBSTITUTION	WHO CLASS*
Metaponto	172 G→A	58 Asp→Asn	3
A–			
Distrito Federal			
Matera			
Castilla	202 G→A	68 Val→Met	3
Alabama	376 A→G	126 Asn→Asp	
Betica			
Tepic			
A	376 A→G	126 Asn→Asp	4
Ilesha	466 G→A	156 Glu→Lys	3
Mahidol	487 G→A	163 Gly→Ser	3
Santamaria	542 A→T	181 Asp→Val	2
	376 A→G	126 Asn→Asp	
Mediterranean			
Dallas			
Birmingham	563 C→T	188 Ser→Phe	2
Sassari			
Minnesota			
Marion	637 G→T	213 Val→Leu	1
Gastonia			
A–	680 G→T	227 Arg→Leu	3
	376 A→G	126 Asn→Asp	
Montalbano	854 G→A	285 Arg→His	3
Viangchan	871 G→A	291 Val→Met	2
Jammu			
A–	968 T→C	323 Leu→Pro	3
Betica	376 A→G	126 Asn→Asp	
Selma			
Chatham	1003 G→A	335 Ala→Thr	3
Loma Linda	1089 C→A	363 Asn→Lys	1
Tomah	1153 T→C	385 Cys→Arg	1
Iowa			
Walter Reed	1156 A→G	386 Lys→Glu	1
Iowa City			
Springfield			
Beverly Hills	1160 G→A	387 Arg→His	1
Genova			
Nashville	1178 G→A	393 Arg→His	1
Anaheim			
Riverside	1228 G→T	410 Gly→Cys	1
Santiago de Cuba	1339 G→A	447 Gly→Arg	1
Andalus	1361 G→A	454 Arg→His	1
Taiwan–Hakka			
Gifu-like	1376 G→T	459 Arg→Leu	2
Agrigento-like			
Kaiping			
Anant			
Dhon	1388 G→A	463 Arg→His	2
Petrich-like			
Sapporo-like			

*WHO denotes World Health Organization; class 1, nonspherocytic hemolytic anemia; class 2, severe enzyme deficiency; class 3, moderate deficiency; and class 4, no deficiency.

64

Since then, five variants were described with similar properties - G6PD Iowa, G6PD Iowa City, G6PD Springfield, G6PD Beverley Hills and G6PD Tomah. All six variants had their mutations in a three amino acid stretch coded by exon X [23]. This part of the protein is conserved, suggesting further that it may be involved in NADP binding.

Mutations are spread throughout the protein, the only significant clustering is of CNSHA variants in exon X, where the NADP binding site is thought to reside. The whole of the protein must intimately co-operate in its functions for an amino acid substitution to have a marked effect on substrate binding, even though the change is topographically far from the binding site. To date, no mutations have been found only in exons III and XIII.

A striking feature is the great variability of mutations. In the last four years, more than 30 different mutations have been found. Many more mutants must exist, since roughly two out of three amino acid replacements are electrophoretically undetectable and others may not result in any amino acid substitution. So the G6PD locus must be the most variable locus in the human genome. There are three possible explanations [27]

1) Mutational- the G6PD gene may have an intrinsically greater than average rate of mutation.
2) Bias in detection- Genes coding for other enzymes are just as mutable, but the products of the mutated genes are less likely to be picked up. The relative ease of detection is reflected by the fact that all Class IV variants have been picked up by electrophoresis, as they are electrophoretically abnormal.
3) Selection- Again mutability may be similar in other genes but the consequent biochemical changes may be less well tolerated and are thus removed by natural selection.

The question arises- how does the mutation alter the function of the enzyme? There is convincing evidence to indicate that mutations alter the stability of the protein. The rate of decline of G6PD differs according to the variant. The half-life of normal G6PD B is about 62 days, 30 days in G6PD Seattle, 8.5 days in G6PD Mediterranean and even less in mutants associated with CNS HA. Decreased catalytic activity alone or in conjunction with accelerated breakdown is also possible. There is no evidence for the mutation leading to decreased synthesis as in thalassaemia. [29]

Characterisation of a new variant

In 1958, Newton et al first described an unusual and totally different clinical syndrome in G6PD deficient subjects. In their words "These patients present the haematological picture of a chronic non-spherocytic haemolytic anaemia with or without specific drug exposure, even though studies on their erythrocytes are comparable to patients who show no anaemia or increased haemolysis except when exposed to specific drugs and fava beans". Since their original report, more than 80 similar cases have been described.

The clinical picture of the propositus is compatible with a diagnosis of CNSHA - mild anaemia associated with reticulocytosis, splenomegaly and acute exacerbations with drug administration or infections. According to WHO recommendations, it is classified as a class I variant. One could argue that the haematological values do not represent the real steady state. Since the investigations were done fifteen days after the crises, the haemoglobin may not have risen nor the reticulocytes fallen to their respective steady states, which may well have been within the normal range. This would be in accordance with a severe Mediterranean -type phenotype, having a normal haematological profile between crises.

CNSHA is usually first noted in infancy, when it is common for it to present with neonatal jaundice as in this case. There is a varying degree of anaemia. In most cases, it is mild. The haemoglobin may even be normal [10] but reticulocytosis is by definition *always* present. There is a tendency for the condition to improve with age as the increased erythrocyte production at puberty has a compensatory effect. The degree of enzyme deficiency may be very severe (less than 5%), but cases have been reported with residual activities in excess of 10%, this being explained by the abnormal kinetics of the enzyme.

Because G6PD deficiency was discovered as a consequence of primaquine administration in 1956, drug induced haemolysis is often considered to be the most common precipitant of haemolysis. This is probably not true. Infections are the most common [3].A critical analysis of data concerning the use of haemolytic drugs in G6PD deficient subjects exposed a discrepancy between the relatively small list of drugs (sulphonamides included) for which there is strong evidence linking them to AHA, and a much longer list of agents for which the evidence is very flimsy. The latter group includes paracetamol which was alleged to have caused a crisis in this patient. It is likely the drug was administered while he happened to have a haemolytic episode or that the real precipitating factor was the infection for which the drug was given. There are cases reported when haemolytic episodes are triggered in the absence of any inciting cause. [7]

Figure 12. Map of G6PD polymorphism in the Mediterranean Bold figures indicate overall frequences (%) of male G6PD deficiency in the respective locations.

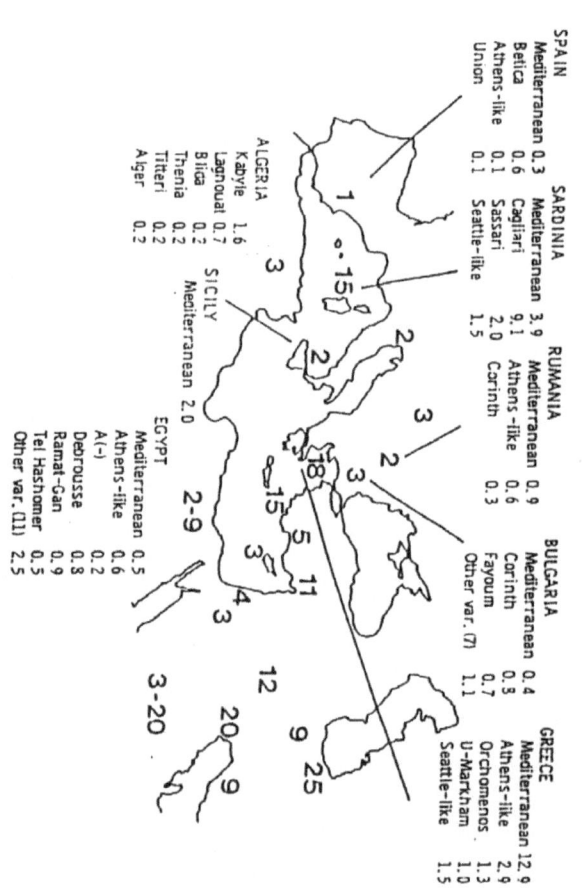

Sardinia has one of the highest rates of G6PD deficiency in the Mediterranean with an average of 15% and peaks of up to 39%[16] and where 8.5% of unexplained NNJ is due to G6PD deficiency [28]. The peculiar altitude -related micro-geographic distribution has long been one of the arguments in favour of malaria selection . G6PD deficiency is more common in villages at sea level than in those at higher altitude [40].Telti is a village with a population of 1,500, 12 km from Olbia in the low lying plains of Northern Sardinia. Ancient Greek colonisation was limited to this area and these communities have been "isolated" for centuries. They are useful for population studies as they closely resemble true Mediterranean isolates.

G6PD in the Mediterranean was thought to be heterogeneous. Biochemical analysis of G6PD deficiency in Sardinia revealed four different polymorphic variants - G6PD Seattle-like, G6PD Sassari, G6PD Cagliari and G6PD Mediterranean. The latter three showed subtle but significant differences in the K_m values and substrate analogue utilisation [18, 42]. It was rather surprising to find that these three variants shared the same mutation in exon VI [16]. Indeed, with very few exceptions, G6PD deficient subjects in the Mediterranean all have the same mutation[8]. Occasionally patients with the common Mediterranean variant have been found to present with CNSHA [10].The reason why some subjects with G6PD Mediterranean have CNSHA, while the majority have a normal erythrocyte life span is not clear. Two possibilities have been suggested – (1) unknown environmental exposures to haemolytic substances inducing what appears to be CNSHA, but is actually merely a subclinical AHA (2) the genetic constitution of the erythrocytes - structure or enzyme - wise. Nevertheless, the exclusion of the Mediterranean mutation in this patient w as a significant step in the project.

There was a single base change from wild type G6PD sequence - a C →T transition at nucleotide 1318 in exon XI, causing an amino acid substitution of leucine to phenylalanine at position 440. The substitution entails no net change of charge and is consistent with normal electrophoretic mobility. The drastic change of an aliphatic to an aromatic amino acid could disrupt the protein structure, affecting its stability adversely.

A single kindred is usually known for CN SHA variants, though quite surprisingly the same mutations have been found recurrently in persons who are not related to each other e.g. G6PD Minnesota, G6PD Marion and G6PD Gastonia all share the same 637 G →T change [8].The mutation of the subject is u nique and as yet undescribed. It has been designated G6PD Telti. The propositus must have inherited the mutation from the mother who was found to be G6PD deficient with 60% residual activity. It remains to be seen if it will be found in unrelated subjects.

Figure 13. An 18 amino acid stretch of exon XI from Human G6PD. Corresponding peptides of Rat, *Drosophilia*, Baker's yeast, *Plasmodium falciparum*, *E. Coli* are aligned. Identical amino acids are designated by a dash.

	432								Tefti ↓						Santiago de Cuba ↓ 449			
Human	Lys	Leu	Pro	Asp	Ala	Tyr	Glu	Arg	Leu	Ile	Leu	Asp	Val	Phe	Cys	Gly	Ser	Gln
Rat	-	-	-	-	-	-	-	-	-	-	-	-	-	-	-	-	-	-
Drosophilia	Tyr	-	-	-	-	-	-	-	-	-	-	-	-	-	-	-	-	-
Baker's yeast	Trp	Ile	Glu	-	-	-	Val	-	-	Arg	-	Ala	Leu	Leu	-	Asp	-	-
P. Falciparum	Val	-	Glu	-	-	-	-	Thr	-	Leu	-	Glu	Cys	-	Lys	His	Lys	-
E. Coli	His	-	Ala	-	-	-	-	-	Leu	-	Glu	Thr	Met	Arg	-	Ile	-	-

71

Some information about the contribution on individual amino acids to the function of G6PD can be deduced from the extent of conservation. Conserved residues are likely to be essential to the function of the enzyme. Mutations of conserved amino acids tend to give more severe disease. Most of the changed amino acids in CNSHA variants are conserved in rat, *Drosophilia*, *Plasmodium falciparum* , *E. Coli* (Mason & O'Brien, personal communication) and yeast G6PD. G6PD Telti is *no exception*. An identical amino acid change in a non-conserved area of exon IX of an unnamed Thai variant is associated with a mild phenotype, as opposed to the severe phenotype of the G6PD Telti mutation in a highly conserved part of the protein.

The G6PD Santiago de Cuba mutation lies just seven amino acid residues upstream from the Telti mutation in a conserved part of exon XI. G6PD Santiago is also associated with CNSHA[45] and has a K_m NADP which is ten times higher than normal. On these grounds, it can be concluded that the region of exon XI, which includes the residues mutated in G6PD Telti and Santiago may be involved in NADP binding.

In conclusion, the analysis of the molecular basis of G6PD variants provides a powerful tool for understanding how the structure of G6PD relates to it s function.

Figure 14 G6PD VARIANTS

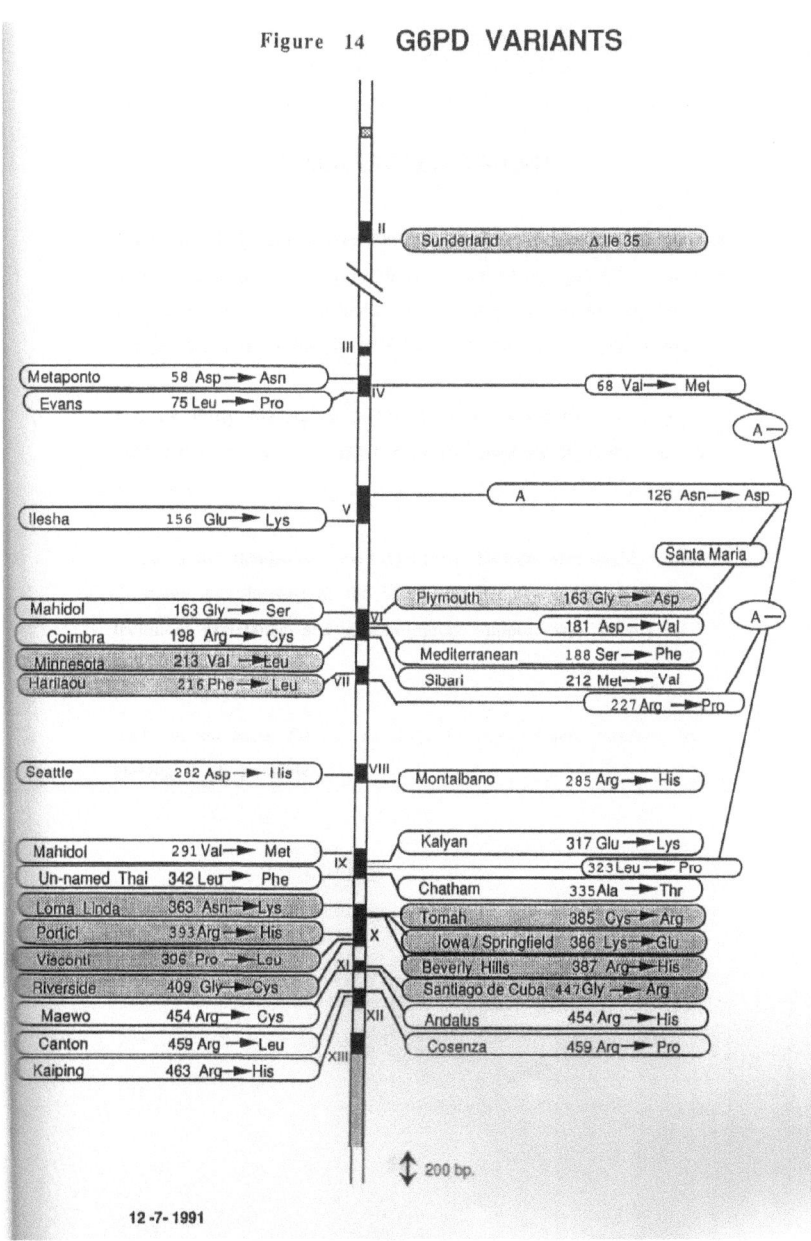

Sunderland	Δ Ile 35
Metaponto	58 Asp → Asn
Evans	75 Leu → Pro
	68 Val → Met
A	126 Asn → Asp
Ilesha	156 Glu → Lys
	Santa Maria
Plymouth	163 Gly → Asp
Mahidol	163 Gly → Ser
	181 Asp → Val
Coimbra	198 Arg → Cys
Mediterranean	188 Ser → Phe
Minnesota	213 Val → Leu
Harilaou	216 Phe → Leu
Sibari	212 Met → Val
	227 Arg → Pro
Seattle	202 Asp → His
Montalbano	285 Arg → His
Kalyan	317 Glu → Lys
Mahidol	291 Val → Met
	323 Leu → Pro
Un-named Thai	342 Leu → Phe
Chatham	335 Ala → Thr
Loma Linda	363 Asn → Lys
Tomah	385 Cys → Arg
Portici	393 Arg → His
Iowa / Springfield	386 Lys → Glu
Visconti	306 Pro → Leu
Beverly Hills	387 Arg → His
Riverside	409 Gly → Cys
Santiago de Cuba	447 Gly → Arg
Maewo	454 Arg → Cys
Andalus	454 Arg → His
Canton	459 Arg → Leu
Cosenza	459 Arg → Pro
Kaiping	463 Arg → His

↕ 200 bp.

12-7-1991

73

REFERENCES

1. Arese P& De Flora A: Pathophysiology of haemolysis in G6PD deficiency. *Seminars in Haem*. (1990) **Vol. 27**, no. 1, pp1-40.
2. Beaconsfield P. Malaria, G6PD deficiency and HbS - *BMJ* (1967) pp 175.
3. Beutler E: Glucose 6 Phosphate deficiency. *NEJM* (1991) **Vol.324** pp 169-174
4. Beutler E: Genetics of G6PD. *Seminars in Haem*. (1990) **Vol. 27**:pp 137-164
5. Beutler E: G6PD deficiency in William's Clinical Haematology (1991) pp 591-605. McGraw-Hill, New York.
6. Beutler E: G6PD: New Perspective. *Blood* (1989) **Vol. 73**; pp1397-1401.
7. Beutler E: G6PD deficiency in the Metabolic Basis of Inherited Diseases. Edited by Stanbury et al (1983). (McGraw-Hill, New York) pp 1630-1645.
8. Beutler E *et al*. DNA sequence abnormalities of Human G6PD variants. *Journal of Biol. Chem* (1991) **vol. 266**; pp 4145-4149.
9. Beutler E *et al*. Molecular heterogeneity of G6PD A -. *Blood* (1989) **Vol 74**; pp 2550-2555.
10. Beutler E *et al*. Biochemical variants of G6PD giving rise to CNSHA. *Blood* (1968) **Vol. 31**; pp131-134.
11. Beutler E *et al*. G6PD Walter Reed: Possible insights into "structural" NADP in G6PD. *Amer. Journal of Haem*.(1986) **23**; pp 25-30.
12. Brown TA: Gene Cloning. (1990) Chapman & Hall.
13. Camardella L *et al*. Identification of reactive lysyl residue labelled with pyridoxal 5'-phosphate. *Eur J Biochem* (1988) **171** pp 485-489.
14. Clark IA *et al*. Activity of divicine in Plasmodium Vinekie – infected mice has implications for treatment of favism and epidemiology of G6PD deficiency. *BJH* (1984) **57**; 479-487.
15. Dacie J. Deficiency of G6PD in Haemolytic Anaemias III. pp 364-417. Churchill Livingstone, 1985.
16. De Vita G *et al*. Two point mutations are responsible for G6PD polymorphism in Sardinia. *Am J Human Genet* (1989) **44**; pp 233-240.
17. Erlich HA. (Ed) PCR Technology (1989) *Stockton Press*.
18. Fenu MP. G6PD deficiency genetic heterogeneity in Sardenia. *Ann Hum Genet* (1982) **46**; pp 105-114.
19. Gaetani GF. Recent developments on G6PD Mediterranean. *BJH* (1988) **No. 63**; pp1-2.

20. Galenser J *et al.* Inhibitory effect of a fava bean component on the *in vitro* development of *plasmodium falciparum* in normal and G6PD deficient erythrocytes. *Blood* (1983) **No 3**; pp 507-510.

21. Heckett, Fuchs, Messing. An introduction to recombinant DNA techniques. (2nd edition) Benjamin/Cummings. Co., California.

22. Hirono A & Beutler E. Molecular cloning and nucleotide sequence of cDNA for human G6PD A-. *Proc Natl Acad Sci USA* (1988) **Vol 85**; pp 3151-3954.

23. Hirono A *et al.* Identification of binding domain for NADP of human G6PD by sequence analysis of mutants. *Proc Natl Acad Sci USA* (1989) **Vol 86**; pp 10015-10017.

24. Howe LJ. & Ward ES. Editors. Nucleic Acid Sequencing. The practical approach series, Oxford University Press, 1989.

25. Hows J & Gordon-Smith EC. Acquired haemolytic anaemias in Postgraduate Haematology, 3rd edition edited by AV Hoffbrand & SM. Lewis. (Heinemann Medical Books).

26. Jeffrey J et al. Characterisation of a reactive lysine residue labelled with acetylsalicylic acid. *Biochem* (1985) **24**, pp 666-671.

27. Luzzatto L & Testa U. Human G6PD: Structure and function in normal and mutant subjects- Current topics in Haem 1; pp 1-70.

28. Luzzatto L & Mehta A. G6PD deficiency in Schriver's Metabolic Basis of Inherited Disease. (1989) pp 2237-2265, McGraw-Hill, New York.

29. Luzzatto L & Battistuzzi G. G6PD - Advances in Human genetics (1985) **14**; pp 217-349.

30. Luzzatto L & Usanga EA. Adaptation of *plasmodium falciparum* to G6PD deficient host cells by production of parasite - encoded enzyme. *Nature* (1985) **313** pp 793-795.

31. Martini G *et al.* Structural analysis of the X-linked gene encoding human G6PD. *EMBO Journal A*(1986) **Vol 5** pp1849-1855.

32. Miller D & Wallman MR. A new variant of G6PD deficiency . G6PD Cornell: erythrocyte, leucocyte and platelet studies. *Blood*(1974) **Vol 44**; pp 323-329.

33. Perbal B. A practical guide to molecular cloning, 1988 Wiley Interscience Publication.

34. Perico MG *et al.* Isolation of human G6PD cDNA clones. Primary structure of the protein and unusual 5' non- coding region. *Nucleic Acids Research* (1986) **14**;pp 2511-1522.

35. Piomelli S. G6PD deficiency and related disorders of the Pentose pat hway in Haematology of infancy and childhood, edited by Nathan & Oski. 3 rd edition. Saunders, Philadelphia.

36. Ratazzi *et al*. G6PD deficiency and chronic haemolysis : relationship between clinical syndrome and enzyme kinetics. *Blood* (1971) **2** pp 205-208.

37. Sanger F *et al*. Cloning in single stranded bacteriophage as an aid to rapid DNA sequencing. *Journal of Molecular Biology* (1980) **143** pp161-178.

38. Sanger F *et al*. DNA sequencing with chain-terminating inhibitors. *Proc Natl Acad Sci USA* (1977) **Vol 74** pp 5463-5467.

39. Sambrook J, Fritsch & Maniatis. Molecular Cloning. A laboratory manual (1982) (Cold Spring Harbour, New York).

40. Siniscalco M *et al*. Population genetics of thalassaemia and G6PD deficiency. Bull WHO (1966) **34:** 379-193.

41. Shallo A *et al*. DKA does not precipitate haemolysis in patients with Mediterranean variant of G6PD deficiency. *BMJ* (1984) **Vol 288** pp 174.

42. Testa U *et al*. Genetic Heterogeneity of G6PD in Sardinia. *Human Genet* (1980) **56** pp 99-105.

43. Vives-Corrons JL *et al*. G6PD deficiency associated with CNSHA granu locyte dysfunction and increased susceptibility to infections. Description of a new variant, G6PD Barcelona. *Blood*(1982) **Vol 59** pp 428-433.

44. Vives-Corrons JL.*et al*. Molecular genetics of G6PD Mediterranean and description of a new G6PD Mutant, G6PD Andalus. *Am J Hum Genet* (1990) **47**; pp 575-579.

45. Vulliamy TJ *et al*. Diverse point mutations in the human G6PD gene cause enzyme deficiency and mild or severe haemolytic anaemia. *Proc Natl Acad Sci USA* (1988) **Vol 85** pp 5171-5175.

46. Watson, Tooze & Kurtz. Recombinant DN A- a short course. Scientific American Books, New York.

47. Williams JG & Patient RK. Genetic engineering. IRL Press 1988.

48. Yoshida A & Roth E. G6PD of malaria parasite, *plasmodium falciparum*. *Blood* (1987) **No 5**; pp1528-1530.

49. Zinder NB & Boeke JD. The filamentou s phage as vectors for recombinant DNA-*Gene* (1982) **19**; pp 1-10.

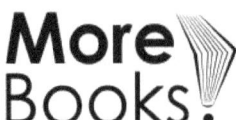
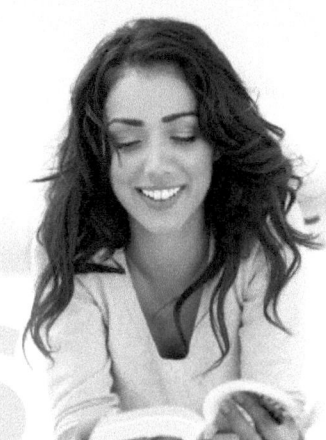

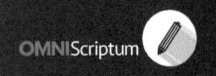

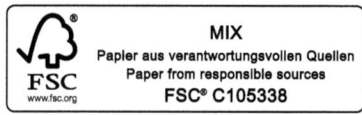